Tudor O. Bompa, PhD

T0280007

TRAINING AND CONDITIONING
FOR
SOCCER

DEVELOP FAST AND AGILE PLAYERS

Meyer & Meyer Sport

British Library of Cataloguing in Publication Data
A catalogue record for this book is available from the British Library

Training and Conditioning for Soccer
Maidenhead: Meyer & Meyer Sport (UK) Ltd., 2025
ISBN: 978-1-78255-281-9

© 2025 by Meyer & Meyer Sport (UK) Ltd.
Aachen, Auckland, Beirut, Cairo, Cape Town, Dubai, Hägendorf, Hong Kong, Indianapolis, Maidenhead, Manila, New Delhi, Singapore, Syndey, Tehran, Vienna

Member of the World Sport Publishers' Association (WSPA), www.w-s-p-a.org

Printed by C-M Books, Ann Arbor, MI
Printed in the United States of America

ISBN 978-1-78255-281-9
Email: info@m-m-sports.com
www.thesportspublisher.com

CONTENTS

PREFACE

For the past few years, we have spent many hours analyzing the current fitness training programs used by most professional soccer teams and have arrived at a not very favorable conclusion. Almost every aspect of fitness training, without the ball, is a program promoted by commercialism. Yet these methods and exercises do not match the physiological requirements of the game. Regretfully, most exercises do not address the physical abilities needed in soccer and are ineffective as seen in the physiological analysis of the game (chapter 1). In addition, you will also notice that there is a clear contradiction between what commercialism is promoting and what the game requires to produce a successful player.

The text is organized into four parts:

Part I is a physiological and methodological analysis of soccer. This analysis will explain the physiological specifics of the game, as well as what the scope of fitness training for soccer should be.

Part II is dedicated to the training methodology needed to develop strength, an essential quality for the development of soccer-specific motor abilities. A detailed discussion will focus on how strength is produced and how the gains in strength will assist the players to develop soccer-specific motor abilities.

Physical training is highly regarded by all soccer professionals who expect their athletes to play a fast game from the first to the last minute. For this purpose, part III is one of the most important sections of the book since it discusses plans and methods necessary to develop game-specific strength, power, speed, agility, and soccer-specific endurance.

Part IV shares soccer-specific training plans and methods that will make you a better and more effective planner. Additionally, we will also discuss an interesting concept of modelling training programs to ready your team and players for future games and tournaments. A long-term guideline for the development of young players and some pertinent examples of training will also be included in part IV.

Soccer professionals have always attempted to find the best methods and training methodology to improve all elements of the game. Therefore, training methodology in soccer is not a novelty. It has existed since 1863, and has evolved from practice, through constant experimentation, to improve technical skills and tactical strategies.

Coaches and soccer professionals have always attempted to discover, from practice, what works and what does not. Some professionals rely on opinions—often good opinions—based on traditions. Others combine experience with scientific finding in exercise physiology, biomechanics, nutrition, and techniques of recovery and regeneration following games and between training sessions. We propose the latter option: a combination of science and methodology to produce the best possible players, techniques, and tactics.

Since strength training is still a confusing concept to some, we would kindly suggest referring to chapter 2, specifically the section titled *How strength and power is produced*, to brush up on the physiology of strength and muscle contraction. In addition, you will discover the physiological relationships between maximum strength (MxS) and power, speed, and agility, and that soccer-specific abilities are impossible to improve without improving strength and power first.

We have used science to improve methodology.

You might be surprised to notice the importance we place on the development of *strength and power*. Please remember that strength is the foundation, the determinant quality that will improve soccer-specific abilities, particularly sprinting speed and agility.

To help you be the best and most successful coach possible, throughout the book we will share with you lots of theoretical and scientific information. Often, we will also offer many examples regarding how to apply a theory in practice, to best serve your players to be as successful as they can be.

An important discussion about exercises is presented at the end of chapters 5 through 8 (called *Exercise Selection*). To us, this discussion is essential since we analyze scientifically and methodically *what works and what does not*. Please analyze this information since it might increase your training effectiveness; select what is best for your players and eliminate what is not.

Please also note that an attempt has been made throughout the book to reduce the size of the text by often using a point format.

Finally, a *law of retention*: for best comprehension, essential concepts of training have been repeated a few times. Our apologies to those of you who might not appreciate it. However, our intent was to best serve your professional interests.

ACKNOWLEDGMENTS

The process of publishing a book is not just the contribution of an author but also the work of many talented and dedicated professionals. I would like to acknowledge those who are part of the team at Meyer & Meyer Sport and whose contributions helped to bring this book together.

First my thanks to Liz Evans, the international program director at Meyer & Meyer Sport. With incredible persistence and efficacy, Liz oversaw the entire process of putting together this book. Without her contribution and dedication, I could not have been very effective in bringing this quality training book to the market and helping those many soccer professionals on their journeys to become the best trainers they can be.

To Anja Elsen, who used her talent in design to lay out this soccer book. Your work, Anja, has been greatly appreciated. A thank you to Anne Rumery and her careful copy edit of the manuscript.

And finally, my thanks to Tom Doherty and Sarah Pursey, who helped to market and promote the book in the US and UK, respectively.

PART I
WHAT IS SOCCER?

For many years, specifically from the 1950s on, many aspects of soccer training, particularly the quality of technical and tactical skills, have been refined to impressive levels. To the delight of millions of soccer fans, the quality of the game has improved not only in the traditional hubs of the world of soccer, Europe and Latin America, but impressive gains were visible in Africa, Asia, Australia, and North America. Highly skilled players with excellent technical qualities elevated their game to impressive horizons. Yet the professionals of the game will never accept the status quo, dreaming, working to produce even better players with superior skills and physical attributes.

Improvement and progress are highly regarded human endeavors, and throughout the content of this book we are humbly attempting to make our contribution to the body of knowledge necessary to elevate the quality of the game of soccer to superior levels. However, before we address the main topic of this work, **soccer-, position-specific fitness training**, we would like to analyze, to refer to some theoretical elements of the physiology of soccer, physical training, and methods used in the sport, to create a foundation that will allow you, our reader, to make an easier connection between what soccer is and why we propose a specific training methodology.

The early chapters of the book refer to training methodology for the improvement of strength, power, speed, agility, and game-specific anaerobic and aerobic endurance. Since physiologically, strength is a determinant physical quality required to achieve a superior level of speed and agility will address this topic first. Then, we will share with you the best methods to train maximum speed and agility, the determinant physical attributes in soccer, followed by the specific endurance. Finally, a condensed discussion about planning will allow us to suggest what and when to train the main abilities during a week (the microcycle).

As the specific training methodology for each motor ability will be presented, a comprehensive discussion will also refer to the selection of exercises. Exercises are essential to make you an effective specialist, to help you target a specific part of the body, the main muscles used in soccer, the **prime movers**. In our case, the prime movers are the calf, knee, and hip muscles.

CHAPTER 1
SOCCER: A SHORT ANALYSIS OF THE GAME

KEY POINTS

- Present State of Training in Soccer
- Time-Motion Analysis
- Training the Energy Systems in Soccer
- Energy Systems: The Scientific Base of Soccer Training
- Energy Systems Analysis for Soccer
- Interaction of Energy Systems
- Restoration of Energy After Training and Games
- Travel Distance

Before discussing how to train we have to find out what we want to train and what soccer actually is. Let us analyze what soccer players have to do during a match. Then, it is much easier to decide WHAT to train and HOW to train them!

Present State of Training in Soccer

Since the early 2000s many elements of soccer training have been visibly altered by the influence of popular trends.

The promotion of new gadgets and training accessories has become more important than the traditional components of the game, the **physiology of soccer**, the dominant physical abilities and bodily functions of the most popular sports of the world.

This is why soccer has become more form (design of training drills) than substance, the physiological aspects of the game. Specific gadgets, accessories, and drills performed with these devices are produced and promoted by some companies as being part of modern training!

Traditional soccer training, where maximum speed, agility, and specific endurance were relatively well trained, nowadays is considered old fashioned, while new gadgets and accessories are promoted as being *the essential part of contemporary soccer training.*

Training accessories have become more important than the physiological effect needed to produce good players. Yet, **without good physiological adaptation, game improvement is impossible, no matter how many modern gadgets you use**. Therefore, contemporary soccer players are just players, not athletes with impressive athletic abilities such as quickness, high speed, powerful take-offs, and the ability to play with high physiological potential in the rhythm of the game for 90 minutes.

The incredible exaggeration of using short duration drills with many gadgets has increased the amount of stress on the ligaments and tendons of the ankle and knees, explaining why there are so many overuse injuries. If you constantly expose your players' legs to many short drills, you should not be surprised that they are anatomically overstressed and experience overuse injuries. Physiologically, the duration of these drills is 4–8 seconds, primarily taxing the phosphagen/alactic energy system but rarely with high intensity. Yet the dominant energy system in soccer is the aerobic system! In other words, *modern training* is clearly missing the physiological target of your training, the aerobic energy system.

Modern training rarely uses drills to enhance aerobic energy system. Please take a stopwatch and time the duration of most drills. Four to eight seconds is far too short to meet the physiological requirements of the game.

Time-Motion Analysis of Soccer

The game of soccer is a very complex, multidirectional, intermittent sport, where all physical attributes are employed in a very competitive environment. The energy base of soccer is aerobic (oxidative), interposed with fast sprints, quick changes of direction and jumps where the energy is supplied by phosphagen (alactic) and glycogen (lactic). The proportions of energy taxed depend on the rhythm of the game, players' position, their physiological potential, game tactics, and size of the field.

Any professional involved in this sport has to understand the abilities soccer players are required to display during the game, and the methods used to improve them. This brief analysis also refers to the source of energy in the following percentage:

15%–15%–70%

In other words, 15% is supplied by the alactic (phosphagen) system, 15% by the lactic acid (glycolytic) system, and 70% by the aerobic (oxidative) energy system (Bangsbo, 1994; Bloomfield et al, 2007; Bush et al, 2015; Dolci et al, 2020). In the case of women's soccer there is a slight difference: alactic 0.5%, lactic acid 19.2, and aerobic 80.3 (Perroni et al, 2019). This reality should make you challenge some of the fallacies of what commercialism calls *modern training*.

- Players run 9-14 km per game (Sarmento et al, 2014), with very little difference between male and female players.
- Players perform 80–90 % of time with lower intensity and 10–20 % with high intensity. During the game players spend their time: standing (4.6 %); walking (14.2 %); jogging (28.1%); running (11.1%); sprinting (4.8%); skipping (9.9 %); shuffling (9.3%); and other (18.2%) (Bloomfield et al 2007).
- Soccer players cover 22-24% of the total game distance at a speed higher than 15 km/hour (km/h), 8-9% at a speed higher than 20 km/h, 2-3 % at a speed higher than 25 km/h (Rampinini et al, 2016).
- A high-intensity run for female elite players is about 30% lower than that for male elite players (Bradley, 2013).
- The duration of a game, including stoppages, is one hour, 36 minutes, and 14 seconds; the actual play time is 59 minutes, stoppages for fouls is 16 minutes, and pauses during the game are 47.19 minutes (Hernandez-Moreno et al, 2011).
- Thierry Henry of France is the fastest soccer player ever with a speed of 39.2 km/h in 1998 (The Healthy Journal, 2023).
- The same source indicates that the fastest woman soccer player was Denise O'Sullivan of Ireland with a speed of 34.5 km/h in 2023.
- The speed of the ball averages 26.4 m/s for men and 22.0 m/s for women.
- During the 2022 World Cup Lionel Messi recorded 87 accelerations and 76 sprints while Cristiano Ronaldo recorded 79 acceleration and 83 sprints (*The Healthy Journal*, 2023).

- Every 90 seconds, a sprint of over 9–14 km/h is performed (Dolci et al, 2020).
- Central attacking midfielders cover the most distance with high speed (Bangsbo, 2014).
- During the game players perform 150–250 brief, intense actions, such as quick changes of direction, jumps, and short sprints (Mohr et al, 2003).
- Players also perform between 1200–1400 changes of directions and more than 600 accelerations and decelerations (Bloomfield et al, 2007).
- Of all the systems of play, the 4-3-3 and 4-4-2 are the most physically demanding and are played with the highest intensity (Dolci et al, 2020).
- Wide and central midfielders cover more distance and perform more high-intensity runs than attackers and central backs (Bush et al. 2015 and Di Salvo et al, 2007) while attackers and wide players perform more sprints (Di Salvo et al, 2007).
- The time spent performing high or very high intensity was 5.6% for strikers, 5.2% for midfielders and 4.9% for defenders (Morgan et al, 2014).
- Defenders tend to use the highest amount of jogging, skipping, and shuffling but less time on running and sprinting (Morgan et al, 2014).
- When high sprints of >24 km/h were considered per game, forwards have run 345 m; external midfielders 314 m; external midfielders 265 m; central defenders 186 m; and central midfielders 167 m (Morgan et al, 2014).
- Total number of sprints per game: short sprints (0–10 m), 7; medium sprints (10–20 m), 48; and long sprints (over 20 m), 45. During the UEFA Cup matches the number of sprints of 10–20 m was 8%, whereas the longest sprints (>20 m) made up 45% of total sprints (Andrzejewski et al, 2013).
- Midfielders and strikers are involved in more athletic actions, such as diving, jumping, sliding, falling, and getting up quickly. Strikers also engage in more physical contact at high intensity (Morgan et al, 2014). This demonstrates why players in these positions need to be physically strong and very good athletes.
- The mean duration of high-intensity sprints (over 21 km/h) in European soccer did not exceed 21 meters (Ade et al, 2016).
- The average work: rest ration for high intensity activities was 1:12 during the game (Di Mascio and Bradley, 2013).

- High-intensity action resulted in 83% of the goals in the German Bundesliga that were performed in the second half of the season (Faude et al, 2012).
- The highest frequency of passes was performed by midfielders (Morgan et al, 2014).
- Compared to other soccer leagues, players from the English FA Premier League and the German Bundesliga have the highest number of headings (Dellal et al, 2011; Bangsbo, 2014).
- There is a lack of information available in the area of strength training. Therefore, it seems that some soccer professionals have not yet reached the level necessary to enable them to equate high-velocity sprinting, jumping, and quick changes of direction with maximum strength and power. This lack of understanding of training needs for soccer has been very well-manipulated by the post-2000 commercialism and some gurus of the internet!

Training the Energy Systems in Soccer

Before discussing training methodology for soccer, first we have to analyze energy systems since the proportion of energy systems dictates the specific content of physical training methodology. From the energy system point of view, the most important objectives of fitness training in soccer are to:

- Improve the specific physiological abilities of soccer to cope with fatigue and to delay the appearance of fatigue. This means the aerobic system is the system inadequately trained in fitness training without the ball.
- Improve physiological foundations to develop maximum speed, to pass an opponent, or to quickly take a specific position in the tactics of your team. To improve maximum sprinting speed also means to train maximum strength, the main ingredient of speed and agility. Have you noticed how strength is trained in the scheme of contemporary fitness training?
- Improve specific endurance to be able to achieve your tactical goals for the entire duration of the game and to facilitate inter-game recovery.
- Prevent injuries via specific strength training (please refer to chapter 3).
- Increase specific physical abilities such as strength and power, the foundations of maximum speed and agility.

Energy Systems: The Scientific Base of Soccer Training

First, a quick review of the dominant energy systems of the body. There are two elements needed for a soccer action to occur:

1. The muscles to contract to perform the skill.
2. The existence of energy, the adenosine triphosphate, or ATP.

ATP is a high-energy compound that allows the release of energy when phosphate bonds are broken. ATP is produced by the three energy systems of the body:

1. The phosphagen system (creatine phosphate), better known by professionals by the term alactic energy system, since it does not produce lactic acid during the activity.
2. The glycolytic system, popularly also called lactic acid, or simply lactic.
3. The oxidative, or aerobic system.

Each system is used to supply energy if the duration of physical activity is performed for a longer period. Let us assume that a player is active, non-stop, for one hour. During the first 10–12 seconds the energy is produced by the alactic (phosphagen) system. When this system exhausts its stores (creatine phosphate stored in the muscles), the glycolytic system, or lactic acid system, is called into action (from 20–90 seconds). From 1–2 minutes through the end of a one-hour activity (in our example), the oxidative/aerobic system is dominant, supplying energy for the entire duration (one hour).

The alactic/phosphagen system primary supplies energy for fast, quick, aggressive sprints and short and quick changes of direction. Both the alactic and lactic/glycolytic systems use carbohydrates stored in the muscles and in the liver in the form of glycogen, therefore, scientifically, it is called the glycolytic system.

The lactic system does not produce energy as fast as the alactic system but has a higher capacity to produce energy for a longer duration (20–90 seconds). As this system is taxed, and demand for energy is still high, the player begins to feel a decrease in the capacity to generate speed due to an increase in fatigue.

The third energy system, the oxidative or aerobic system, produces energy at a slower rate, but for a longer duration than the first two systems. Because energy production by this system relies on the breakdown of carbohydrates and fats, energy production is slower but lasts for hours. Table 1.1 illustrates specific elements of energy systems: the rate of producing energy, the fuel used for each system, and the rate of recovery for each energy system after it has been used.

Table 1.1 The three energy systems that supply energy for soccer

Energy system	Rate of producing energy	Duration	Fuel used	Duration of rest interval/ recovery time per unit of activity
Phosphagen (alactic)	Very high	1–12 seconds	Creatine phosphate	1:12–1:20
Glycolytic (lactic acid)	High	20–90 seconds	Blood glucose, glucose stored in the liver	1:3–1:5
Oxidative (aerobic)	Low	2 minutes– 2 hours, or longer	Glucose stored in muscles and the liver; fat; protein	1:1–1:3

Based on information from Ekblom 1986, Bangsbo et al 2006, Bompa and Haff 2009, Dolci et al 2020.

The duration of rest interval for phosphagen/alactic system, 1:12, means for one unit of time (i.e., 10 seconds) the rest interval is 12 times higher (120 seconds or 2 minutes). The duration of rest interval for glycolytic/lactic acid is 1:3, meaning that for a duration of one minute of activity the rest interval is three minutes. The duration of rest interval for oxidative/aerobic is 1:1, meaning that for an activity of five minutes at lower intensity work, the restoration time is also five minutes.

Interaction of Energy Systems

The three energy systems do not act independently but rather interact in a specific sequence to generate the necessary energy to sustain physical work, from the shortest burst of energy (aggressive sprints) to enduring an exhausting game. Coaches' and instructors' comprehension and imaginative use of these systems has led to the improvement of training science and methodology over the years.

As illustrated in table 1.2, the three energy systems interact to produce the energy required to support physical work. The interaction of the energy systems is directly related to the duration of the activity. Keep these guidelines in mind when planning and designing different types of training to target the individual energy systems.

Table 1.2. Percentage contribution of energy systems for technical, tactical, and physical training

Activity duration	Alactic	Lactic acid	Aerobic
5 s	85%	15%	0%
10 s	50%	40%	10%
30 s	15%	65%	20%
1 min	10%	40%	50%
2 min	5%	25%	70%
4 min	2%	18%	80%
10 min	1%	9%	90%
30 min	–	5%	95%
1 h	–	2%	98%
2 h	–	1%	99%

Based on information published by Bangsbo et al, 2006; Bompa, 2006; Powers et al, 2008; Perroni et al, 2019.

Although all three energy systems must be well trained with and without the ball, the aerobic system provides most of energy during the game, being also essential for a strong finish of each half of the game. In addition, a well-developed aerobic system facilitates a faster recovery after games and between training sessions.

Table 1.3 Time needed for the restoration of the three energy systems

Recovery process	Minimum	Maximum
Restoration of muscle phosphagen	2 minutes	5 minutes
Repayment of alactic oxygen debt	3 minutes	5 minutes
Repayment of the glycogen oxygen debt	30 minutes	60 minutes
Restoration of muscle glycogen: After intermittent activity After prolonged nonstop activity	2 hours to restore 40% 5 hours to restore 55% 24 hours to restore 100% 10 hours to restore 60% 48 hours to restore 100%	
Removal of lactic acid from the muscles and blood	10 minutes to remove 25% 25–30 minutes to remove 50% 60–75 minutes to remove 95%	

Compiled based on information from: Fox, 1984; Bangsbo, 2006; Bloomfield et al, 2007; Powers and Howley, 2011; Dolci et al, 2020; Perroni et al, 2019.

Energy System Analysis for Soccer

Soccer is an intermittent, high-intensity game. During the course of a game, players perform everything from sprinting, jogging, striding, walking, kicking, and jumping to making agile turns and quick changes of direction.

Generally, the higher the level of play, the higher the energy demands and overall stresses experienced during the game. However, playing in a high-intensity game is possible only if players dedicate adequate time to training and only if coaches design training around the position-specific requirements of the game.

The ergogenesis (proportions of energy systems used in sports) for men's soccer has been estimated at 15% alactic, 15% lactic, and 70% aerobic, and 0.5 % alactic, 19.2 % lactic and 80.3 aerobic for women's soccer (Perroni et al, 2019). Furthermore, a breakdown of energy system by position as well as the position-specific motor characteristics required in soccer is suggested by table 1.4. Please note the differences in energy systems and motor abilities between most players and especially for mid-fielders and sweepers.

Table 1.4 Ergogenesis per position in soccer

Position	Ergogenesis
Goalkeeper	Alactic: 100%
Sweeper	Alactic: 30% Lactic: 30% Aerobic: 40%
Fullback	Alactic: 20% Lactic: 30% Aerobic: 50%
Midfielder	Alactic: 10% Lactic: 20% Aerobic: 70%
Forward	Alactic: 20% Lactic: 20% Aerobic: 60%

Compiled based on information from: Ekblom ,1986; Bangsbo, 2006; Bompa, 2006; Thorpe et al, 2017; Perroni et al, 2019; Bompa and Sarandan, 2023.

As already known, soccer players use all three energy systems during the game: alactic, lactic, and aerobic. With sprints in soccer lasting an average of 4.5 seconds, a good portion of the energy is supplied by the alactic system. When these sprints are frequently repeated during the game, phosphagen stores are depleted. Now the energy demanded is supplied by the lactic acid system.

Low glycogen levels among players are very common at halftime, and players often completely deplete their entire glycogen stores by the end of the game. However, if the demand of the game is low, postgame glycogen levels may remain at 15 to 20% of pregame levels. This is not the case for highly disputed games. Therefore, for optimal glycogen replenishment, to support their need for energy, players must consume diets rich in carbohydrates. This is even more important for players with a busy schedule (i.e., two or three games per week), since diminished glycogen stores reduce the capacity to play with high intensity for all games.

The glycogen restoration is not immediate. About 60% is restored in 10 hours, while full restoration takes about 24 to 48 hours—one reason soccer teams should not play more than two games per week. Ignoring these physiological realities could harm the players, resulting in high levels of fatigue, staleness, injuries, and even overtraining.

The institutions planning the schedule of soccer games should also consider the energy availability for all these games, levels of exhaustion, and the time necessary to replenish the energy. A good planning of soccer games will be highly respected by players and team owners. Equally important is to show some sensitivity towards the players and coaches regarding the stress they are exposed to and their need to relax, recover, and regenerate between games.

Travel Distance and Game Intensity

The distance covered per game is position-specific and may depend heavily on the rhythm and pace of the game. Highly competitive games tend to be more physically and mentally demanding. In some of these highly contested games, top players have been known to cover distances of about 10 km. Midfielders, the so-called engines of the team, usually cover more distance than other players—an average of 11 km per game. The longest distance run by a soccer player so far was a French player, Henry Duquette, who in 1989 covered 15 km in a single game and currently holds the record (The Health Journal, 2023).

Next in line are the forwards, who average 9.5 km per game, followed by fullbacks, averaging 8.5 km per game. Considering their specific tactical responsibilities within the team, one should not be surprised that, except for goalies, sweepers cover the least amount of ground—an average of 6 km per game. Of course, these values vary from game to game, depending not only on the pace of the game and levels of fatigue but also on the skill level of the players and varying climatic conditions.

Table 1.5 The average distance covered (km), mode of movement, and physiological demands for soccer players (by position), expressed as percentages per game's intensity

Position played	Average distance covered (km)	Mode of movement					Physiological intensity per game	
		Walking	Jogging	Striding	Sprinting	Other	High	Low
Forward	9.5	2.5	4.0	1.25	0.8	0.95	40%	60%
Midfielder	11.1	2.8	5.0	1.5	1.0	0.8	50%	50%
Fullback	8.5	2.5	3.5	1.1	0.6	0.8	30%	70%
Sweeper	6.0	2.1	2.5	0.6	0.5	0.3	30%	70%

Compiled based on information from Ekblom, 1986; Bangsbo et al, 2006 and 2014; Bompa, 2006; Bloomfield et al 2007; Hands and de Jonge, 2020.

Of the total distance covered, individual players performed at about 10% at maximum speed, with sprints varying from 10 to 40 m. If sprints and striding/ cruising are considered together, higher-intensity running approaches 2.5 km. The rhythm of the game, the conditioning level of the players, and the air temperature and humidity are important factors affecting performance intensity. Games in hot or humid conditions tend to be played at lower intensity, but they experience increased levels of physiological stress.

The higher the league or level of play, the higher the game's intensity. The intensity of a game is also reflected by the amount of weight loss (generally through increased perspiration) experienced by players during a game. Games played at a faster pace or rhythm or in higher temperatures or humidity tend to elicit greater weight loss. In temperate climates, such as those in northern Europe and the United States, weight loss per game can range between 1.5 and 2 kg per game. However, in warmer climates, such as those in the southern United States, South America, Africa, southern Asia, and southern Europe, dehydration levels can reach up to 5 kg during high-intensity games. This level of dehydration can severely affect speed and especially endurance (Thorpe et al, 2017).

Another indicator of game intensity is the lactic acid concentration in the blood, which can range from 8 to 12 millimoles. Games of lower intensity yield lower levels of lactate concentration.

Finally, heart rate can also be an accurate indicator of game intensity. Heart rate values for high-caliber players can often exceed 180 beats per minute (bpm) during a game. Depending on the pace of the game, the heart rates of highly involved players can rise to between 184 and 186 bpm 12 to 16 times in a single game, demonstrating the high levels of intensity to which a soccer player may be exposed (Bangsbo, 2014).

A Friendly Message to Fitness Instructors in Soccer

Strength and conditioning (S&C) coaches are enthusiastic professionals with diverse backgrounds. Some have a four-year college degree; others completed a certificate program from an online course or, at best, from a one-week seminar. The emphasis in these seminars is on exercises, though often the ones promoted in these seminars do not address the training physiology of soccer. Without a good comprehension of training physiology, S&C may not be able to maximize their talents. If you are a soccer coach seeking a strength and conditioning coach for your players, or if you want to become a strength and conditioning coach, keep in mind the following:

- Some S&C programs focus on teaching as many exercises as possible. However, quantity does not mean high-quality programs.
- Some S&C coaches have good information regarding exercises, but there is more room for the improvement of soccer physiology. Exercises without improved physiological adaptation to training will never assist you in increasing players' physical potential.
- On the contrary, a lower number of exercises with a higher number of repetitions and sets results in higher soccer-specific physiological adaptation.
- Exercises are necessary only as a means to target the prime movers (the essential muscles needed to perform certain athletic/technical moves). Local physiological benefits, however, come from the training program, from the number of repetitions and sets.
- Knowledge of exercise physiology, particularly in the area of neuromuscular systems, is determinant in becoming a successful S&C coach. Do you want to be the best S&C trainer? Spend more time on sports physiology.
- Understanding the fundamentals of sport science and science-based training methodology is essential to effective training.

- The methodology of training young players, which is essential for the formation of future top players, appears to be an area of neglect and in need of diligent revamping. Improving youth soccer begins with information from biology, growth and development during the childhood and teen years, energy systems training, methodology of developing age-group motor abilities, sport psychology, and nutrition.
- Strength training is one area of training that is often misunderstood and improperly organized. Some of the gadgets and training methods promoted as effective are not validated by science (physiology, biomechanics). Maximum strength (MxS) increases the recruitment of fast twitch (FT) muscle fibers, the fibers so essential for the improvement of power, speed, and agility.
- Strong muscle contractions that bind together actin-myosin filaments are at the foundation of developing power, speed, and agility.
- Power, maximum speed, and agility increase only after a well-developed strength and power training. Therefore, it will be an error to expect your players to be fast and agile before you expose them to strength training, particularly maximum strength (MxS).
- Players are able to increase speed and agility only when capable of applying high amounts of force against the ground during the propulsion phase of the running step.
- If knowing a selected set of exercises is a necessity, knowledge of exercise physiology, particularly in neuromuscular physiology, is determinant in being a successful S&C. Do you want to be a successful trainer? Learn the fundamentals of exercise physiology!
- Only sports science and science-based training methodology can make you excel in the profession you love.

Have you ever timed the duration of the training drills that abound in contemporary fitness training programs without the ball? If you do that, you will find that the vast majority of the drills have a duration of only 4–8 seconds! In other words, the energy used in these drills is alactic (phosphagen) and you are targeting the energy systems that **supply only 15% of the energy required during a game of soccer!**

Technical coaches demand a **high rhythm** of the game throughout the 90 minutes. However, the training methods used in contemporary fitness training for soccer are far from being a guarantee that coaches' expectations will ever be achieved.

Have you watched what is trained in contemporary fitness training for soccer? When are the energy systems trained to ensure a high rhythm of the game (lactic and aerobic)? If your fitness training without the ball is not addressing the dominant energy systems, how can you expect your players to be effective in a game with a duration of 90 minutes? With this type of training, you are not justified in demanding high and continuous rhythms of the game from your players.

A friendly suggestion to the stressed coaches:

- Maintain a positive team atmosphere of calm, confidence, and realistic optimism.
- Monitor each player's health status regularly.
- Create a relaxing atmosphere for yourself as well.
- Remember: you are also exposed to a high degree of stress.

Commercial Trends in Training: Just a Consideration

Commercialism is the new game in town! It opened the doors to an elusive training methodology that in many cases does not meet the professional rigors of science and methodology. New gadgets are promoted by some sports industries with the promise that they improve speed and specific endurance, agility and strength, in spite of the fact that the resistance used during some exercises is so low that improving strength is an impossibility.

Resistance bands and stability balls are promoted to improve balance, strength, and proprioception, which improves athletic performance. Just because a player steps on a stability ball, it does not mean the result will be the improvement of leg strength. On the contrary, our suggestion for more sport-specific training is to examine the multitude of exercises backed by science, including our proposed training programs (parts II and III). Regarding the development of strength, power, maximum speed, and agility, a trainer must incorporate those exercises proven to improve player performance.

We strongly suggest that every training enthusiast participates in the process of improving the quality of training by adhering to the fundamentals of exercise physiology, biomechanics, and methodology of training.

Fitness training in soccer is already dominated by commercial trends, in spite of the fact that some suggestions are clearly contradicted by the physiology and methodology of soccer. Ultimately, the onus is on the expertise of the soccer professionals, who have made soccer the most popular sport in the world. Therefore, please analyze the difference between scientific information and the promotions made on the market and draw your own conclusions.

> Constant progress, from high technology to soccer training, is a desirable human endeavor, but to promote inadequate training concepts is not. This is why some of the newly promoted methods and gadgets in soccer training do address mostly the form or architecture of a drill, without improving the fitness level of players or the physiological needs of soccer, such as cardiovascular, respiratory, and the neuromuscular systems.

Conclusions

The above analysis of the soccer game has two major purposes:

1. To penetrate into the most intimate elements of the game, particularly the physiological details of soccer training, and
2. knowing this information, to motivate you to organize your overall fitness program to ready your players for what is expected of them during the game.

Please consider that the most important aspects of training you have to dedicate time to are:

*   The time spent on high intensity was around 5% per game (Morgan et al, 2014; Ade et al, 2016; Dolci et al, 2020). Yet, almost all the time dedicated to fitness training without the ball is of short duration (4–8 seconds) and which is supposed to be of high intensity! Why spend most of the time for

fitness training on an activity that is only 5% of the total time of a soccer game? When is the remaining 95% trained?

- Forty-five percent of total sprints are for >20 meters. How often do S&C instructors train the players to be effective for that distance?
- Distance travel has to be duplicated in training to ensure your players will be ready to be an effective player not only in the first half of the game but also for the second part.
- It is necessary to comprehend the proportions of energy systems (ergogenesis) required during the game and to train them during the preparatory phase. In this way, by training the players to cope with fatigue during the workouts, your players will be ready to reproduce it during the game.
- The dominant energy system in soccer is aerobic: 70%. The balance is 15% for the phosphagen (alactic) and the remaining 15% comes from lactic acid (glycolytic energy system). Therefore, concentrate on the physiology of soccer training and the dominant energy system used.
- A friendly suggestion to both the technical and fitness coaches: for the best benefit of your team, you have to closely cooperate in every aspect of training. Soccer coaches should try to learn and effectively understand the scope of fitness training with but also without the ball. You should know what is effective for your players and what is not. Always scrutinize the type, methods, and exercises used in fitness training without the ball. You should also analyze the work done by your players and quantify it. Evaluate it. Both types of soccer training, with and without the ball, result in fatigue. Evaluate the level of fatigue and apply the best methods to assess it and recover between training sessions and after games.

CHAPTER 2
THE SCOPE OF PHYSICAL TRAINING IN SOCCER: MAKING FAST, AGILE, AND RESILIENT PLAYERS

KEY POINTS

- The Scope of Physical Training in Soccer
- Selected Pitfalls in Contemporary Soccer Training
- We Need Fast Players!
- Muscle Structure and Functions
- Strength Training and Neuromuscular Adaptation
- How Strength and Power Is Produced

Chapter 1 familiarized you with the specific elements of the physiology of soccer. Now we can begin discussing physical training and the development of the dominant motor abilities in soccer, starting with strength, power, speed, and agility, and ending up with game and position-specific endurance.

The scope of physical training in soccer, and the entirety of part II of this book, is not just to illustrate how to develop the physical abilities of soccer players but to also suggest how to transform a player into an authentic athlete. An athlete with superior physical abilities, such as strength, will always make a player faster, more agile, and more capable of playing an aggressive game.

Most players on the pitch are just players, and they play the game only with the potential they currently have. When soccer is played by better athletes, the game looks different, with superior qualities, such as powerful technical moves and fast penetrations into the opponent's side on the field, faster and longer sprints, more abrupt changes of direction, and an improved rhythm of the game.

The quality of the game also improves as a result of applying the methodology of energy systems training, from alactic to lactic and aerobic systems. The use of these three energy systems must be planned in such a way that will allow the coach to alternate energy systems and facilitate recovery and regeneration between training sessions and games.

Strength training should not be considered just as a method to lift heavy weights, or to build big muscles! In soccer, strength has to be considered as the foundation of all soccer-specific motor abilities.

In a very condensed form, the main objectives of strength training are:

- to overcome resistance (e.g., gravity, opponents),
- to use specific training methodology to increase power, speed, and agility and maximize quickness, and
- to use a specific methodology to improve speed endurance, muscle endurance, or the capacity to perform long duration, nonstop, technical, and tactical actions throughout the game.

Selected Pitfalls in Contemporary Soccer Training

Our intent in this book is to discuss science-based training concepts and to offer better and more efficient, practical training methodology and methods. The following list summarizes an analysis of the present state of training in soccer:

- The determinant physical abilities in soccer are power, speed, agility, and soccer-specific, position-specific endurance.
- Most programs for developing the physical attributes in soccer have good intentions, but they miss the mark. Often, they are the victims of misleading and inappropriate methods promoted by the latest trends in fitness training, which are unrelated to soccer training.
- Most contemporary fitness drills in soccer are organized in bouts of 4-8 seconds! Why? Because some of the gadgets, accessories, and drills currently used in soccer are that long! However, the duration of the game is 90 minutes, and the main energy used during the game—70% of the total—is supplied by the aerobic system. This is why we have to ask the question: how can you train the physiological needs of soccer (70% aerobic, 15% anaerobic, and 15 % anaerobic) with drills that tax just the alactic energy system? When and how are the other energy systems taxed in soccer, lactic acid and aerobic, trained? Did you ever compare soccer

training methodology proposed by commercialism with what science and methodology is suggesting?
- The energy requirement of the game is a scientific reality, but some strength and conditioning coaches overemphasize the alactic system.
- Strength, power, maximum speed, and agility are also trained with some exercises of short duration, targeting the phosphagen energy system. However, some fitness coaches often neglect developing maximum strength (MxS), power, maximum speed, and game and position-specific endurance.

Most coaches are always looking for young players who are talented and fast. Some players are equipped with the abilities needed in soccer: speed and power. Others are not. Genetics also play a role in players' abilities—that is the proportions between muscle fibers type: the white fast-twitch (FT) fibers or the red slow-twitch (ST) fibers.

A coach wants a player who has a higher proportion of FT muscles. Simply, this player is naturally suited for soccer as they will be fast and agile. When a young player inherits a higher proportion of ST fibers, his or her talent is mostly for aerobic-dominant, endurance sports, since the red fibers are very effective in supplying oxygen to the working muscles. Marathoners are a great example of the importance of ST muscle fibers: 82% of total muscles fibers are ST, whereas 18% are FT muscles. In the case of soccer, the proportion is visibly different: 58% ST vs. 42% FT (Costill et al, 1976; Van Someren, 2006).

But players and coaches shouldn't despair if a young player who may not be genetically talented at soccer shows potential because this person still has a chance to become a good player by improving power, speed, and quickness. The best way trainers can help them develop is by exposing them to strength training (part III). Using good, sport-specific strength-training exercises and stressing maximum strength (MxS) can increase the force of the player. As a result, the player's capacity to generate higher force—and consequently increased speed and agility—is facilitated by activating a higher number of FT muscle fibers. This increased physiological potential will translate into the capacity to apply higher force, making the player faster and more agile.

One might then expect that fitness training for soccer must be very specific to match the physiological makeup of this game. The reality, however, is different, since the majority of fitness training in contemporary training without the ball is not soccer specific for two reasons:

1. Despite what a trainer may plan to develop power, speed, agility, and reactivity, most drills are low speed, low intensity, the exact opposite of the expectations of some strength and conditioning (S&C) instructors. To achieve this objective, drills have to be high intensity to enable the player to recruit FT muscle fibers in action. Without recruiting these fibers, a player cannot be expected to improve speed, agility, and quickness.
2. Often the duration of a drill is far too short to have any effect on the development of soccer-specific lactic acid and aerobic endurance.

Strength Training and Neuromuscular Adaptations

When a player is exposed to strength training, the body is progressively adapting via structural and physiological changes. These functional changes are directly proportional to the intensity/load, quantity/volume, and frequency of training. The resulting benefit from quality strength training is the load (intensity), particularly in speed- and power-dominant sports. Higher loads invariably result in increased strength. As the player's capacity to overcome resistance increases, he becomes stronger, directly improving power, sprinting speed, and agility. As explained in the following chapters, the adaptation to high loads translates into increased recruitment of the FT muscle fibers. The higher the recruitment of FT muscle fibers, the higher the improvement of speed and agility, essential physical qualities in soccer. Nobody can increase power, speed, or agility without first improving strength.

Since the 1900s, the early years of strength training, many strength-training enthusiasts asserted that strength was determined mainly by a muscle's size, or the cross-sectional area. This is why strength training for sports was directly influenced by bodybuilding methodology: to build big muscles. Although, to some degree this is visible even nowadays, strength-training research since the 1970s (by authors such as Sale, Schmidtbleicher, Duchateau, Zatsiorsky, Clark, and Weyand, etc.) has focused on the neural component of the physiology of strength. Furthermore, the essential role of the nervous system in strength training for sports was well documented by Broughton (2001).

As already mentioned, the load in strength training is an essential contribution to the type of strength and its neuromuscular adaptations. This is why when S&C trainers decide on the type of strength training to incorporate for their players, they have to consider that there are two specific types of training loads, each with their own specific physiological adaptations and benefits:

1. Lower loads, below 70% 1 repetition maximum (1RM), improve intermuscular coordination, or the ability of the prime movers (the muscles that perform the dominant technical actions) to learn to work together in unison and with good coordination and to perform a skill with lower resistance (high-frequency coordination, medium-speed sprints, and agility).
2. Heavy/high loads, over 80% 1RM, result in improved intramuscular coordination, or the capacity to recruit the highest number of FT muscle fibers in the action. Training programs intended to increase power, reactivity, sprinting speed, and agility must use the intramuscular coordination, maximum strength, and power methodology. If they don't, do not expect visible athletic improvement...

Physiology of Muscle Structure and Its Functions

From simple walking to very complex athletic action, every movement is produced by contractions of the muscles, often called the engine of the human body.

The capacity of muscles to produce force is genetically determined and largely depends on the muscles' size and cross-sectional area, length, and number of muscle fibers involved in the action. S&C trainers and technical coaches should know that strength training, especially the MxS methodology, does increase the thickness of the active muscles and the force of contraction, their power, sprinting speed reactivity, and agility (Schmidtbleicher, 2019; Dorn et al, 2019; Duchauteau et al, 2021).

All muscles of the human body have two types of fibers, red, or slow twitch (type I) and white, or fast twitch (type II). Slow-twitch fibers are best for aerobic-dominant sprints. They are slow to fatigue, have a smaller nerve cell (innervates 10-180 muscle fibers), and are recruited during long-duration activities. Fast-twitch fibers are best for anaerobic-dominant sports. They are quick to fatigue, have a larger nerve cell (innervates 300-500 muscle fibers), and are recruited during speed, power, and agility actions. The contraction of fast-twitch muscle fibers is obviously more powerful and faster than that of its slow-twitch counterpart.

The muscle fibers are grouped together to form a motor unit, the motor neuron and the muscle fibers it innervates. Every motor unit contains thousands of muscle fibers that contract when a soccer action is performed. Altogether, athletes are equipped with thousands of motor units and muscle fibers.

The reaction of a motor unit directly depends on the load it has to overcome. If a player must perform a calf press with a heavy load, such as 80% of 1RM, fast-twitch muscle fibers are quickly stimulated to contract and perform the exercise. The same physiological action occurs when a player has to react quickly, accelerate, make a quick changes of direction (agility), or kick a ball. In these instances, the player must recruit a fast-twitch muscle fiber. All these characteristics can be directly improved by MxS strength training methodology.

How Strength and Power Are Produced: A Brief Scientific Demonstration

High sprinting abilities and quick changes of direction are determinant in many aspects of the game, particularly during tactical plans intended to surprise the opposition players. This subchapter must be considered a very important part of the book since it will discuss:

- how muscle force is produced,
- how strength training, specifically the maximum strength (MxS) method, will increase the capacity to recruit in action a higher number of muscle fibers,
- how important strength and power are for the development of fast and agile players,
- that strength training does not build huge size muscles,
- the relationship between the number of muscle fibers involved in action and the speed of the player,
- how only strength training can improve the capacity of the smallest elements of a muscle, the myosin and actin filaments, to contract with higher force and thereby increase speed and agility,

- that without a higher propulsion, push-off phase of the running step, a player will never be able to increase speed, sprinting, and jumping capabilities,
- that the propulsion phase can be increased only by using a good methodology of strength training, particularly MxS, and
- finally, how ineffective some exercises used in contemporary soccer training modes are. Try to evaluate them. You might be surprised to note that many of them are not useful for training soccer players. Most of them do not address the prime movers, particularly for the legs, and consequently, are inefficient use of training time.

This is why the following discussion regarding the physiology of **muscle contraction** is so essential to comprehend and **apply in soccer training**. Fast sprinting and quick agility actions are produced by the capacity to increase a muscle's strength, and to apply it against the ground to quickly run in the desired direction.

To best understand how strength training enhances athletic performance or improves your game-specific physical qualities, you need to know the science behind it; specifically, you should understand **the physiology of muscle contraction**, known as the **sliding filament theory** (Huxley and Niedergerke, 1954; Enoka, 2015; Schmidtbleicher 2019). For more information on the slide filament theory please refer to figures 2.1 through 2.3 and their accompanying text.

Figure 2.1 illustrates the structure of a skeletal muscle, from the tendon—where it originates from—to the muscle fiber, ending in the smallest element of a muscle, the muscle filaments. These two **muscle filaments are the essential elements of muscle contraction** which are called actin (thin filament) and myosin (thick filament).

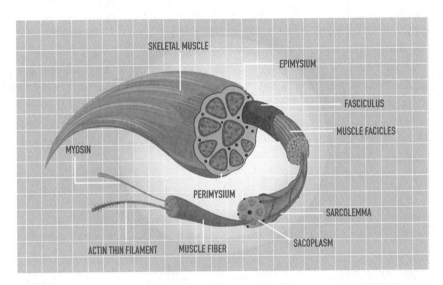

Figure 2.1 An illustration of a muscle: from the attachment of the tendon to the bone to the myofilaments.

When a muscle contracts, the myosin heads (crossbridge, the extensions from myosin towards the actins) are activated, binding them with the actin and pulling against it (see figure 2.2). This action results in the overlapping of myosin with actin, pulling the myosin against the actin, and, as a result, producing a muscle contraction (shortening of the muscle), which generates the force necessary to produce an athletic action.

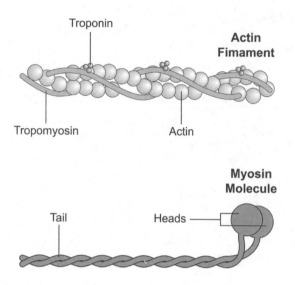

Figure 2.2 The sliding filaments of muscle contraction: The engine that produces force, maximum speed, and abrupt agility.

The overlapping and sliding of actin and myosin produces the necessary force to overcome gravity, the weight of an implement, or the force of an opponent. Force produced by this sliding action is also at the base of moving fast or with agility. **The stronger the muscles, the stronger the propulsion phase of the running step, and the faster the player's sprinting ability and agility.**

Figure 2.3 illustrates the size of a myosin filaments of a player who has been exposed to MxS. The myosin filament is much thicker, and the number of cross bridges is higher, demonstrating the typical adaptation for a player involved in MxS training. Such a player is naturally equipped to generate higher force, a quality that positively influences the player's sprinting speed and agility.

Myosin heads (cross-bridges)

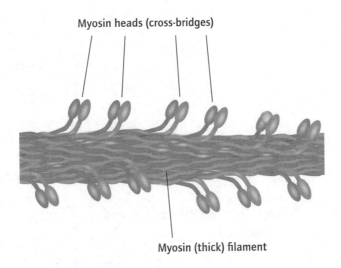

Myosin (thick) filament

Figure 2.3 The thicker myosin filaments of a player exposed to MxS.

None of these athletic abilities are possible without first developing MxS. The result of MxS training is the increase of the number of cross bridges and the thickness of the myosin filament, that, in turn, results in a stronger pull. Stronger pull always means higher generation of force (figure 2.3). The thicker the myosin, and the higher the number of myosin heads (cross bridges), the higher the capability of the player to produce force. What is the athletic consequence? A stronger, faster, and more agile player!

To produce faster, more agile players, you need to expose them to a progressive and well-organized strength-training program that develops thicker myosin and a higher number of myosin heads; in other words, train for MxS (see chapters 3-5). If, on the other hand, you will only apply some traditional training methods (i.e., 5-10 repetitions of short and fast sprints), you will improve speed and agility only during the first few weeks of training. Furthermore, if training for MxS is absent from your power and speed-training program, the result will be a plateau. Toward the end of the playing season, it can even decrease the quality of speed and agility. The same situation will also happen to a player throughout their career (i.e., improvement during the early years and plateau after).

Conclusions

The most important element discussed in this chapter is the physiology of muscle contraction, particularly the sliding filament theory. Your comprehension of this scientific reality will allow you to demonstrate, not only to yourself, but to other professionals, the fact that strength training, as proposed in this book, will not result in increasing big muscles, but rather will increase just the myosin thickness and the number of cross bridges. The thicker the body of the myosin filament and the higher the number of cross bridges, the more powerful the pull of the cross bridges against the actin. The result is quite predictable: increase the force of muscle contraction and, consequently, increase the sprinting speed and the quickness of an agility drill.

The sliding filament theory is of determinant importance to imagine what can happen to a soccer player if the player is exposed to a real strength training program. Please remember that most soccer moves and skills require a specific type of strength, power, or agility. High power means quickness, high sprinting speed, and agility. Please do not forget that MxS training should always be part of your plan. If you overlook it, you'll have serious difficulties producing fast and agile players and might even fail to achieve your team's objectives.

MxS training in soccer is also important because it increases the force capability of your player since heavy loads (80–95%) increase the recruits in action of high number of the powerful fast-twitch muscle fibers, making a player faster and more agile.

PART II
TRAINING METHODOLOGY TO DEVELOP STRENGTH: THE SOURCE OF ALL SOCCER-SPECIFIC ABILITIES

Chapters 1 and 2 gave us the opportunity to review the physiological foundation of soccer, particularly, during the time-motion analysis of the game, energy systems, as well as the importance of strength training to produce the best players. Each coach must have a good understanding of what happens inside of a muscle exposed to strength training. As discussed in part I, the necessary road to a good physiological adaptation is a progression of training methods that will result in the development of the dominant abilities in soccer: power, speed, agility, and specific endurance.

Throughout chapters 3–9 we concentrate on discussing the most effective training methodology, with practical, applied methods, to ensure that everything we will refer to will have a soccer-distinctive aura.

The organization and content of part II follow a clear physiological progression (Schmidtbleicher, 1984 and 2019; Sale, 1986; Weyand et al, 2000; Bangsbo, 2006; Van Someren, 2006; Bompa and Haff, 2009; Von Lieres et al, 2020; Dolci et al, 2020; Ekstrand, 2021):

- Adaptation (A) to strength training has a dual scope: to build the base for the MxS phase to follow, and to prevent injuries.
- Maximum strength (MxS) has the physiological scope of strengthening the prime movers, the muscles performing key technical skills and athletic moves, and increasing the ability to recruit in action the highest number of muscles fibers to produce the fastest athletic moves.

- Power, speed, and agility can reach the highest standards only if MxS is developed first. The scope of power, speed, and agility training is to increase the discharge rate and the quickness of muscle contraction, since these abilities can reach the highest level only if the muscle fibers contract with the highest force and rapidity.
- Soccer-specific endurance training (chapter 9) will be based on the energy systems training (alactic, lactic, and aerobic) and used and maintained throughout the duration of a league games. **Remember:** what your players improved during the preparatory phase has to be maintained during the league games. If you neglect it, your team will pay the price towards the end of the league games.
- In chapter 9, specific endurance training will be a practical yet clear example of how to use energy systems theories to train soccer-specific physical abilities and to organize training and recovery process between training sessions and after the games.

Throughout these discussions we will compare what works and what does not, along with what is effective training methodology and what is not! A similar approach will be used in our discussion regarding the selection of exercises. This discussion will be based on *research findings and scientific evidence to* propose the best methods and exercises.

Progression to Develop Soccer-Specific Abilities Prior to League Games

Before discussing the methodology to develop soccer-specific motor abilities, the highly regarded high sprinting and agility qualities, we have to discuss its progression, the periodization you have to organize to improve these dominant abilities prior to starting the league games.

Figure *a* illustrates the annual plan for league games in two parts of the world of soccer: Argentina, Brazil, Uruguay, and the other countries in the southern part of the South American continent (at the top of the chart) and Western Europe, the second row. For each of these rows we have listed the months of the year (according to schedule of the league games) so that below it, we can suggest how to plan training phases and the periodization (the sequence of development of each motor abilities important in soccer) of strength and other soccer-specific abilities.

For instance, since in Brazil, Argentina, Uruguay, etc., the league games start in April, the months of February (F) and March (M) are planned for preparing, to ready the players for the league games (April–December). The month of January (J) is reserved for players' removal of fatigue, rest, and recovery, a transition (T) from one season to the next.

The following rows illustrate how strength, speed, agility, and soccer-specific endurance are periodized. The specifics of training for each physical ability are discussed below, in chapters 3–9, referring to both training methods and exercises, as applicable to soccer.

Argentina, Brazil, Uruguay	F	M	A	M	J	J	A	S	O	N	D	J
Western Europe	J	J	A	S	O	N	D	J	F	M	A	M
Training phase	Prep		League Games									T
Per. strength/ power	A	MxS	Maintain force									A
Per. of speed	S, M, L		Maintain									/
Per. of agility	S, M		Maintenance									/
Per. Spec. end.	Aerobic	AL/LA	Maintain specific endurance									Aerobic

Prep = preparatory phase; T = transition towards the next season/vacation, remove fatigue, recovery, relaxation; A = adaptation; MxS = maximum strength; Periodization of speed: S = short distance (10–15m), M = medium distance (20–30 m), L = long distance (35–40m); Periodization of agility: S = short duration (5–10 seconds), M = medium duration (10–20 seconds); AL = alactic; LA = lactic acid energy systems training.

Figure a Guidelines for periodization of soccer-specific abilities during the annual plan. Please note that the calendar dates might not correspond. The possible discrepancy might be of 2–3 weeks difference. (For example, in Western Europe, the preparatory phase might start at the end of June and the league games might start in the second part of August.)

Specific remarks are necessary regarding the periodization of each physical abilities, starting with strength training, the essential physiological ingredient to produce high sprinting speed and agility in soccer. It is impossible to reach high standards in speed and agility without the contribution of strength. However, to reach your athletic objectives, to develop maximum speed and agility, you need first to develop maximum strength (MxS) and power, abilities that require slightly longer time for the body to adapt to it.

Part II, which is dedicated to discussing the development of strength is divided into two phases:

1. adaptation to strength training, a progressive adaptation (A) to increased strength training loads (chapter 3), and
2. maximum strength (MxS) where heavier loads are employed to increase players' capacity to apply higher force against the ground to improve maximum speed and agility (chapter 4).

At the end of part II, we will share with you the results of a research study led by Dr. Sarandan (chapter 5) where the purpose was to compare two training programs:

1. a contemporary training program, used in almost every soccer club and country (program proposed by commercialism), and
2. a training program based on science and top training methodology, the training concepts discussed and suggested in this book.

We will appreciate your perusal of the study; you may draw your own conclusions from it.

CHAPTER 3
TRAINING METHODS FOR DEVELOPING
GAME-SPECIFIC STRENGTH

KEY POINTS

- Strength Training and Its Determinant Role in Producing Fast and Agile Players
- The Neuromuscular Strategy to Improve Soccer-Specific Physical Abilities
- Adaptation to Strength: The Foundation of Strength Training for Soccer
- Injuries and Their Causes
- Injury Prevention
- Ligaments and Tendons: A Sensitive Issue in Soccer
- Program Design
- Maximum Load Method: The Source of Speed and Agility
- Training Methods for the Adaptation Phase
- Exercise Prescription

As an important sporting ability, strength is the foundation of most other motor abilities (figure 3.1). You will never be able to improve speed and agility without using strength, particularly maximum strength (MxS), as the foundation. Chapters 3–8 offer the possibility of exploring what strength is and its relationships with power, sprinting speed, and agility.

Strength training should not be considered just as a method to lift heavy weights or to build big but slow muscles. Definitely not! In the case of soccer, strength has to be considered as the foundation of all the soccer-specific motor abilities: power, sprinting speed, and agility (figure 3.1).

In a very condensed form, the main objectives of strength training are:

- to overcome resistance (gravity, opponents),
- to improve strength to ameliorate specific running-based actions, such as sprinting speed and agility,

- to justify the types of strength physiologically,
- to use specific training methodology to increase power, speed, agility, and quick feet,
- and high frequency in your legs' actions,
- to use a specific methodology to improve speed endurance, or the capacity to perform
- longer-distance sprints, and an effective transition from offence to defense, defense to offence,
- and a high rhythm of the game, and
- to employ the methodology of MxS for the purposes of recruiting the highest number of fast-twitch muscle fibers to improve the capacity to apply highest force against the ground to enhance high speed and agility during the game.

Misconceptions Regarding Strength Training

Have you ever heard the saying: We don't need strength in soccer? While some professionals do accept that strength training can be beneficial to produce strong and fast players, others still adhere to the following misconceptions.

- **Strength training increases muscle size!** Increasing muscle size is just a normal adaptation to training. If you expose your players to short and fast sprint training, from childhood on, over time you will notice that your players' legs have gained in size but also in speed and ability to quickly change directions. Therefore, a slight increase in size is just a natural occurrence, a physiological adaptation. As muscles become stronger, speed will also increase for the simple reason that an increase in speed is possible only when muscles become stronger. Additional proof is presented in the following chapters.
- **Strength slows down our players!** Yes, strength can either increase or decrease a player's physical potential, depending on the training method you are applying. If you expose your players to bodybuilding, a training method that always results in increased muscle size, but not in the quickness

of muscle contraction, then you will likely slow down your players. Why? Because muscles always adapt physiologically to the training method you expose your players to. Contrary to the bodybuilding method, the MxS methodology increases the force and speed of muscle contraction that results in increasing running speed, making your player faster and capable of quickly change directions. In reality these are the essential physical attributes in soccer. Not bodybuilding or trendy exercises.

Do you want to be fast and agile? Plan effective MxS and power training.

Strength Training: Its Determinant Role in Producing Fast and Agile Players

In sports training, strength is rarely used in its pure form or in isolation, excepting weightlifting and power lifting. Similarly, strength training in soccer does not refer to how big your muscles are or how much weight you can lift. On the contrary, strength in soccer is the main ingredient to produce the soccer- and position-specific speed, agility, and speed endurance (figure 3.1). Without this physical component the development of power, speed, speed endurance, and agility will be impossible. Furthermore, in order to maximize the benefits of MxS for your players you have to also select the best exercises that correctly target the prime movers, specifically the gastrocnemius and soleus muscles, the real engines of sprinting speed and agility.

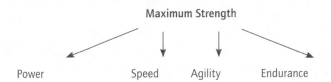

Figure 3.1 The role of strength, the main ingredient in the production of power, speed, and agility.

A simple analysis regarding the interrelationships between maximum strength (MxS), speed, and endurance results in the following combinations:

- **Maximum strength (MxS)** combined with **speed** results in improved **power** and **agility**, or the capacity to perform dynamic and explosive athletic actions on the pitch, or in reduced space in offence and defense. High propulsion force during short sprints, jumps, abrupt and quick agility, and specific athletic actions performed by central and full backs, forwards, and wings are impossible to achieve without the contribution of powerful leg muscles.

- **MxS/power** combined with prolonged **speed** results in **speed endurance**, visible in sprints longer than 30 m, or in longer duration tactical actions, often performed by midfielders, during both offence and defense.

The Periodization of Strength for a Traditional Soccer Team

Soccer players and their neuromuscular systems must be trained to adapt to the specifics of the game and according to the training program designed by the coach and S&C trainer. As players are exposed to an organized training program, their neuromuscular systems also adapt to the training they are exposed to.

For improving soccer-specific physical attributes, strength training must follow the concept of periodization of strength, targeting game- and position-specific physical qualities (part III).

This discussion also addresses the positive and negative aspects of most training methods and exercises as well as how to apply them to your training programs. To assist players in improving soccer-specific abilities that directly depend on strength, you are invited to peruse the organization of an annual strength-training plan or a cycle of games in a soccer league.

Training phase	Preparatory			League games	Transition
Neuromuscular strategy	Adaptation	Increase recruitment of FT fibers	Increase discharge rate of FT fibers	Maintain the ability to recruit and discharge FT fibers	Recovery and regeneration, balance development
Periodization of strength	Adaptation	Increase force (MxS)	P/S/A	Maintain force, speed, and agility	A
Training benefits	Muscle adaptation to strength	Increase muscles' capacity to improve force	Improve maximum speed and agility	Maintain the improvement level of specific abilities	Rest, recovery

A = adaptation to strength training, FT = fast-twitch, MxS = maximum strength, P/S/A = power, speed, and agility

Figure 3.2 The periodization of strength for soccer from the early preparatory phase through the end of the league games or. Please adapt the duration of each phase according to your own conditions.

The annual training plan (figure 3.2) for a traditional soccer team: preparatory, league games, and transition, where the scope is to achieve the highest performance during the league games. Immediately following that, there is the periodization of strength with its phases:

- Adaptation, or three to four weeks progressively increasing strength training using lower loads. Younger and lower league players may prolong this phase to five to six weeks, depending on their own abilities. Longer adaptation means longer time to ready the players for the next phase.
- The second phase is an essential one: the development of MxS, where the scope is to increase players' strength as per their potential. By using heavier loads, the players will be able to increase the thickness of myosin filaments and the number of cross sections so that the recruitment of FT muscle fibers will increase and MxS will improve; this is essential for the development of sprinting speed and agility
- As the league games approach, the scope of training becomes more game-specific by increasing the discharging rate of the FT muscle fibers (the quickness of contraction), resulting in improved power (P), speed (S), and

agility (A). This training objective can be achieved in approximately three to four weeks, but preferably over a longer time (six weeks). The quickness of muscle contraction can be increased by using lighter equipment, such as medicine balls, that allow the players to visibly increase the application of force.

Adaptation to Strength: The Foundation of Strength Training for Soccer

Let us take each training phase to discuss the main elements of strength training and to also offer some training examples. In this chapter we will discuss the foundation of all types of strength training, and in the next chapters we will share with you the methodology of MxS followed by power, speed, agility, and soccer-specific endurance.

Adaptation (A) for soccer can be best comprehended by using this simple analogy: Have you ever watched how tall buildings are built? From the foundation up to the roof? Do you know that the solidity of the foundation dictates the number of floors you can build?

We can also use this analogy for the methodology of producing top players: to start with a strong foundation, move to the adaptation phase, and progressively reach the highest level of strength, power, agility, maximum speed, and sport-specific endurance.

The adaptation phase is essential for building a strong fitness base of progressive adaptation and, as a result, will ensure injury-free soccer players. As you plan your A training for the following league games, you should consider the following training concepts:

- The scope of the adaptation phase is to adapt, ready, and prepare the cardiorespiratory and neuromuscular systems for the next league games.
- To best train the neuromuscular system, specifically the muscles, ligaments and tendons, you have to use progressive training loads, from low to medium, as suggested next in our training programs for the adaptation training phase.

- The obvious scope of adaptation for strength training is to ready and adapt the neuromuscular system to tolerate heavier strength-training loads that will be used during the MxS phase.
- Do not push! Allow your players, especially young players, to progressively adapt to medium loads and be ready for the MxS.
- Develop an overall and specific flexibility, particularly for ankle, knees, and hips.
- Develop the aerobic and anaerobic endurance to increase players' working capacity, to tolerate fatigue and psychological difficulties, and be an efficient player at the end of each half of the game.
- Remember that adaptation also means readying your players for the entire season with psychological preparation.
- Qualities such as perseverance, fighting power, resilience, and discipline create the best inter-player social relationships, and above all, allow you to be a controlled fighter for your team and yourself.
- Since injuries are the cause of many disappointments, it is important to understand the causes of injuries before discussing prevention strategies.

Injuries in Soccer: Causes and Suggestions

Prior to discussing the specifics of a training program for the adaptation phase, we would like to justify why this type of training is so important in soccer: prevention of injuries.

Soccer is one of the sports that experiences many injuries, especially in children. Most of them occur in the lower limbs: ankle sprains, anterior cruciate ligament (ACL) tears, meniscus injuries, groin adductors and hamstring strains. Recent gimmicks used in fitness training in soccer should also raise the question of inappropriate physical training (strength, specific endurance, and flexibility training). In addition, the use of ineffective exercises and gadgets is one of the reasons that the number of overuse injuries has increased in the past few years.

In Spain, the same injuries have reached a rate of 81% (García-Fernández et al, 2017). A study of 10 years of high school soccer injuries concluded that sports professionals show the need for injury prevention programs (*British Journal of Sports Medicine*, March 2017).

The same source also refers to the situation in Italy, where there are more injuries per hour of practice in soccer than in rugby! Yet rugby is a more physical game than soccer. Why is that? Could it be that rugby players have better strength-training methodology and, as a result, are more able to prevent injuries than soccer players? Is soccer such a dangerous sport? Or, might it be those certain types of training in soccer, specifically strength, power, and flexibility, are inappropriate?

Remember: Only strength training (adaptation and MxS) can ready your players to tolerate high mechanical stress on muscles and joints.

A brief analysis of injuries in soccer shows that many have common causes:

- Since professional players are highly paid, they will do everything to be able to maintain that status, including risky actions during the game.
- Game schedule is year-round. Players' vacations are rarely longer than two to three weeks.
- Professional players are under constant stress, including mechanical and anatomical stress, particularly on the ankles, knees, groin (abductor muscle group), and low back.
- To improve sprinting speed in soccer, you have to first increase players' strength, particularly MxS. The best training solution is to plan an anatomical adaptation (AA) phase prior to training MxS and before the beginning of the league games. In this way your players are exposed to an injury-prevention phase, a very effective training plan to keep your players healthy.
- Be sure to pay equal attention to strength training for quadriceps and hamstrings, since an imbalance between them can often lead to injuries. between,
- Some soccer professionals rarely adhere to a strategy of injury prevention. The most exposed joints and muscles which suffer are the foot, ankle, knee joints, and groin muscles. This reality is even more visible since strength training as part of contemporary training has adopted a high array of ineffective exercises. Since the load in many such exercises is low, the mechanical stress encountered during the game is often higher than the force players use in training. Not surprisingly, the outcome is leg injuries.
- The mechanical stress encountered by players in training, particularly on ankle and knee joints, is really high. You must consider whether your players

are being properly exposed to such loads in their strength training program and whether they are able to overcome this stress by doing the following:

» Walking: 2.8 times higher than own body weight (OBW)

» Jogging: 3.6 times OBW

» Leg press: 4-6 times OBW (D'Lima et al. 2012)

Not surprisingly, most injuries are recorded in August and January, prior to the beginning of the new league games (Jan Ekstrand, M. Hagglund, M. Walden, 2011). Furthermore, 92% of soccer injuries affect four major muscles (Jan Ekstrand, MD, UEFA Medical Committee, 2012-2019):

• hamstrings: 37%

• adductors (groin): 23%

• quadriceps: 19%

• calf (gastrocnemius-soleus): 13%

Most injuries to hamstrings and groin occur because of inappropriate strength training (particularly MxS), using low loads and leaving the muscles untrained to withstand the mechanical stress they are exposed to during the game. The low rate of injuries to the calf muscles is explained by the fact that these muscles are the strongest of all skeletal muscles in the human body.

Finally, based on a study of 10 years (2001-2010) by Hagglund et al (2013), Ekstrand et al, (2023), and Hagglund (2023), the number of incidents of injuries have visibly increased as of 2013, but particularly from 2016 on (figure 3.3).

Could it be that contemporary training is superficial and not concerned with injury prevention methodology? Flexibility training seems just like a simulation, whereas strength training is a pretense.

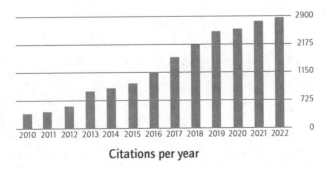

Figure 3.3 The rates of incidents of injuries per year (adapted from Hagglund, 2023).

Consider the data in figure 3.3:

- Should owners of professional soccer teams pay more attention to the type and quality of a fitness training program?
- Do S&C trainers and soccer coaches know that a successful sprinting speed training should start with an adequate strength-training program? That high sprinting speed is achievable only if your players can apply higher force against the ground? A low force application means lower sprinting speed.
- Soccer coaches and S&C trainers should evaluate training programs used in sprinting events in track and field. After all, both sports want to produce fast athletes.
- Track sprinters are strong athletes capable of applying a very high force against the ground and the starting block: 174 kg for the front leg and 168 kg for the back leg (Francis and Bompa). Generally, sprinters in track are so much faster than soccer players because they have much stronger muscles, ligaments, and tendons. How do soccer players compare with the track sprinters in those areas? When strength training for soccer is sport specific, players will be faster and more resilient, and there will be fewer injury incidents.
- Scientific research claims that the highest incidents of injuries in soccer occur during games (Ekstrand et al., 2023). A possible reason for this is that many of the latest training methods and exercise trends are not appropriate for the sport. The mechanical stressors players experience during games are often much higher than those experienced through training with low weight loads and low application of power.
- Most injuries in soccer occur in the ligaments and tendons, not at the muscle level, (Hagglund and Walden, 2016). Yet, coaches and S&C trainers rarely address this issue, particularly the methodology of injury prevention via a well-organized strength-training program.
- Tendons are important in transmitting the force of the working muscle. If tendons are improperly trained, they cannot transmit force and cannot withstand the high mechanical stress specific to high sprinting speed, jumping, and agility. Ankles are among the most neglected joints, both for strength and flexibility training. Unfortunately for most soccer players, the degrees of plantar and dorsiflexion are very low. Ankle rigidity opens the door to injuries. A good strength-training program can be part of your injury prevention strategy. In order to prevent injury, the ankle joint (tarsals

and the metatarsals) and ligaments have to be strengthened with calf press exercises and high pressure dorsi flexion (chapter 8), side-to-side movements, as well as rotations against resistance with heavy loads.

- Strength training for the preparatory phase is often too short and superficial. Following the periodization of strength training method ensures that there is adequate time spent training as well as a focus on power, agility, and springing speed.

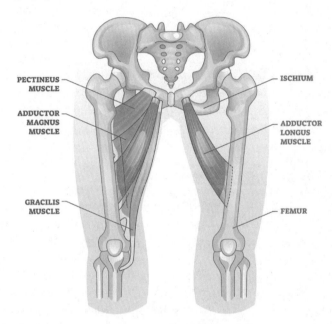

Figure 3.4 The adductor muscles are frequently susceptible to injuries in soccer.

Injury Prevention

Strength training and injury-prevention programs for some professional teams and players are often overlooked. Furthermore, some fitness programs tend to neglect the training of ligaments and tendons because the adaptation phase training is inappropriate, very short, or nonexistent. Therefore, an injury prevention program has to be organized for all players, beginning with the preparatory phase. This is equally true for team owners where injury means a financial loss in their investments in highly paid players. An examination of fitness training for soccer is overdue.

The warm-up should be seen as an important activity to prevent injuries. A good warm-up prepares players for a good training session and should follow this well-known progression: jogging, calisthenics, overall stretching, running/ simple agility drills.

Watching a warm-up for a training session for track sprinters would give soccer trainers a good idea of what would be effective in their players' warm-ups.

To be effective, injury prevention training for soccer must concentrate on the following two motor abilities:

1. **Flexibility training** for the main joints in soccer (ankle, knees, and hips [coxofemural]) should also incorporate the groin and the hamstrings. Maximum angles or degrees of flexibility required during the game should be the minimum angles or degrees trained during workouts. Consequently, flexibility should be trained at the highest acute angles possible during each training session, mostly at the end of the warm-up and at the end of the training session.
2. **Strength training**, the force (load) a player applies against the ground to generate high sprinting speed and abrupt agility must be the minimum load used during the MxS phase training. If you do not follow this concept, sprinting speed in soccer may stagnate or fail to improve, and the incidents of injuries for your players will remain high.

The force (load) used during high-velocity running during the game, say 70 kg (154 lb) during the push-off phase, has to be the minimum load used during strength training for the leg and calf press. More realistically, the load for the calf press can easily surpass 120–150 kg. For the calf press, top players should have the potential to use even higher loads (> 200-250 kg or more).

This is a very safe and effective method of preventing injuries. The loads in strength training are usually quite low, and as a result, application of force against the ground during the push-off phase is low as well. If you want your players to run faster and to change direction quickly, you have to improve the force of their prime movers (the push-off, the propulsion phase of the running step).

When you train the calf (calf press), you also prevent injuries by strengthening ankle ligaments and tendons.

Prevent Injuries Rather Than Treat Them

The quickness of a player relies not only on the force of the propulsion phase. Equally important is to improve the quickness of knee flexion, the recovery phase of the running step, via the improved strength of the hamstrings. Gluteal-fold strength, where the upper hamstrings meet the buttocks, is essential for the pawing or brushing phase of the running step. Most hamstring injuries are localized near the upper hamstrings, the muscle-tendon junction. The reverse leg press is a more effective exercise for strengthening the upper hamstrings than the leg curl. This exercise can be done also be done on a hammer reverse leg press machine.

Ligaments and Tendons: A Sensitive Issue in Soccer

Any soccer skill is the result of mechanical work performed by muscles. More importantly the force of muscle contraction depends on the actions of two muscle filaments: actin-myosin coupling. To perform work, the muscles have to contract and transmit their force to the bone via a tendon; as a result, the limb moves to perform a sporting skill. Therefore, if a tendon is a transmitter of force, the ligaments keep the anatomical integrity of a joint intact.

Please remember:

- The better your strength-training program, the stronger the ligaments and tendons.
- The stronger the ligaments, the more stable the joints.
- The more stable the joints, the easier it is to prevent injuries.
- Well-trained, strong tendons can withstand great mechanical stress. If the strength capability of tendons and ligaments is inappropriate, they may become a limiting factor for performance, a weak link in a stronger chain. As a result, every time these connective tissues are exposed to high mechanical strain, they may produce anatomical discomfort or even injury.

S&C professionals should remember that unlike muscle tissue adaptation, which takes a shorter time, connective tissue (ligaments and tendons) adaptation often takes several weeks, up to twelve (McDonagh and Davies, 1984; Bohm et al, 2015; Monte et al, 2020). This time requirement justifies why we suggest a longer A phase for most players, especially for the younger players. The adaptation training must focus not only on strengthening the muscles but also on fortifying the connective tissues, such the Achilles tendon (figure 3.5).

Fast and strong runners always have a very powerful gastrocnemius muscle, inserted on the heel, on the calcaneus bone. The injury-prevention strategy of any soccer coach must be the improvement of the gastrocnemius's strength that directly results in the strengthening of the Achilles tendon. Furthermore, strong tendons always have a larger area where the tendon is attached to the bone. In the case of the Achilles tendon, the insertion area is 65 mm2 or more (Enoka, 2015). The larger the size of attachment of the Achilles tendon, the better insurance against injuries

Note: For strengthening the Achilles tendon and its insertion you can use the following exercises: short and powerful sprints, running stairs, skipping rope, calf press, hill raise, and plyometric exercises such as low jumps on the toes and ball of the foot, low jumps (one and two feet) on the spot, jumps over low hurdles,

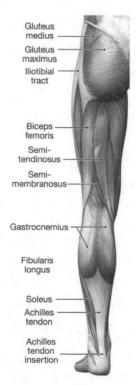

Figure 3.5 The calf with the gastrocnemius, soleus, and insertion of the Achilles tendon on the calcaneus bone and the heel.

To best understand why gastrocnemius is called the king of sprinting, the strongest skeletal muscle of the human body, please consider the following physiological features:

- It has, by far, the highest number of muscle cells: 1,120,000. As a comparison, the darling of most fitness instructors, the quadriceps, has only 1,934 cells. For any forward propulsion, push-off actions, it can recruit the highest number of muscle fibers of all the skeletal muscles of the human body. As such, it can generate the highest force of all muscles. Please remember this equation: increased force = high velocity
- It has the highest number of end plates (~2,000) that innervate muscle cells. The higher the number of innervated (stimulated) muscles, the higher the force and sprinting capabilities of a player.
- The Achilles tendon can transmit the highest maximal force, 510 kg, from the gastrocnemius to the foot (Enoka, 2015; Blazevich, 2021). When the foot can apply higher force against the ground, the player can reach higher velocity and changes of direction.
- For all soccer-related leg actions performed on the ground (sprinting, jumping, agility), gastrocnemius is the muscle with the highest contribution. Strengthening this muscle via A and MxS should be a major training goal, enabling players to be fast and quick in changing directions and performing agile motions.

To sum up how to prevent injuries:

- Always use good technique when performing soccer skills and actions.
- Use proper fitness training equipment.
- Do not overdo it.
- Educate players regarding injury prevention.
- Do not take risks. High risks can result in injuries.
- Always do a good cool-down and stretch thoroughly.
- Severe injuries may start from a small one.
- See your doctor for any discomfort you might feel.
- Make sure you are completely healthy before you train again.

Adaptation Training Phase: A Progressive Build-Up as the Base for Strength Training

Gains in strength do not occur overnight but rather cumulatively, over time, and in a specific, physiological sequence. For good organization and maximum effectiveness, strength training for soccer follows a planning concept called **periodization of strength** (figure 3.2). The term *periodization* comes from the word period, meaning period of time or training phase. In training methodology, the periodization of strength has five training phases, each with clear training goals (figure 3.2).

Strength training must start with the adaptation (A) phase to ensure a progressive increase of the loads, or a progressive adaptation; use this phase as a strategy for injury prevention. In addition, the adaptation phase is also preparing the player for the next phase: MxS.

Normally, all players follow a yearly program intended to enable peak performance during league games based on a proper physiological foundation, including strength training. Such a program must be well-planned and periodized. This is true of strength training. Strength can be refined through various methods and exercises that can create the desired final product: soccer-specific strength, power, speed, and agility.

Strength training should be performed throughout the annual plan, following the concept of the periodization of strength; this will ultimately transform strength into a soccer- and position-specific physical ability. In the following chapters we discuss the best training methods, go into specific details, and finish with an overall annual plan (chapter 10). This discussion also addresses positive and negative aspects of most methods and exercises, and how to apply them in your training programs.

Training Methods for the Adaptation Phase

For soccer, strength training must be a long-term proposition: from childhood (U12) up through the highest professional teams. Soccer players reach their highest performance level not after four to six weeks of a strength-training program but rather during the league games, which come weeks after the adaptation (A) phase. Therefore, the goal of the adaptation (A) phase is to progressively adapt the muscles, especially their attachments to bone (tendons), so that they can cope more easily with the heavier loads used in the ensuing training phases. As a result, the overall training load must be increased without causing the athlete to experience much discomfort.

The simplest method to consider for the adaptation (A) phase is a simple group of exercises called circuit training (CT), developed in post-WW2 England at Leeds University (Morgan and Adamson, 1959). CT provides an organized structure, alternates muscle groups, and can be used not only to develop the foundation of strength for future training phases but also to develop nonspecific cardiorespiratory endurance by combining strength with some simple endurance activities. Incorporating the cardio program into a circuit is compatible with strength training used during the adaptation phase.

The selection of exercises for CT may involve several muscle groups of the body, including the prime movers. First decide which muscle groups you want to target, then choose the specific muscles you want to target. For the highest training effectiveness for soccer, select from the following limbs and muscle groups:

- **Legs (ankles, hips, and knees).** Concentrate on toe raises, hip thrusts, hip flexion, knee flexion, and knee extension. Concentrate also on the foot motions on the sagittal plane, such as eversion (lifting the inner side up) and inversion (lifting the outer side up). The strengthening of the foot using the above motions against resistance represents an injury-prevention strategy for the foot.
- **Core muscles (back and abdominals).** Concentrate on trunk extensions and rotations for the intervertebral muscles, trunk extensions for the lumbar, and flexions and rotations for the abdominals. A strong core assures overall stability and support of the body. Remember that the trunk is a fulcrum, transmitting force from the legs to the arms and from the arms to the legs. This is why it has to be strong to support most exercises and actions performed during contests.
- **Arms and shoulders.** Concentrate on flexions and extensions, pull and push, adductions, abductions, and so forth. Players may use their own body weight, light to medium loads, medicine balls, simple apparatus, and training machines.

During CT you can use a wide variety of implements such as body weight, medicine balls, light implements, dumbbells, barbells, and strength-training machines. To ensure a good progression CT may be short (6-9 exercises), medium (10-12 exercises), or long (13-15 exercises) that can be repeated several times, depending on the number of exercises involved and players' physical potential. The more exercises, the fewer circuit repetitions. The number of circuits can be 2-3 for long circuits and 3-4 for the shorter ones. The number of reps per station should start higher (e.g., at 20) and decrease over time (e.g., down to 8-10) as the load is progressively increased prior to the beginning of the MxS phase. The rest interval can be 30-90 seconds between stations and 1-3 minutes between circuits.

Total workload during the adaptation phase should not cause the players pain or great discomfort. Remember progression? Players should help determine the amount of work to perform. Circuit training is a useful, though not magical, method for developing the foundation of strength during the adaptation phase. Simpler training methods can be equally beneficial if they alternate the muscle groups and have a positive, physiological benefit for your players.

Program Design

This chapter and the following ones suggest training programs, which may be used or adapted based on your own conditions, players' physical potential, and phase of training.

Adaptation training may be used from the first few weeks of this phase. Select the workstations according to the muscle groups you want to target based on the equipment available. Players should follow a certain progression, depending on their classification and training background.

Younger players with little or no strength-training background should start with exercises using their own body weight or lower loads (e.g., medicine balls, small dumbbells, empty barbells). Over time, they can progress the load using heavier medicine balls, loaded barbells, and strength machines. However, the prime movers (the muscles primary used in soccer) should also be targeted as the engines for speed, agility, and technical skills.

The load and the number of reps and sets should be individualized and work up to the point of feeling either slight or actual discomfort. For slight discomfort, read uneasiness. Discomfort, on the other hand, refers to the threshold at which the player is maintaining good technique but must stop the exercise due to eventual soreness. Similar differences apply to the number of stations per circuit. Because young players must address as many muscle groups as realistically possible, they use more stations, and their circuits are longer. Advanced players can reduce the number of stations to focus on exercises for the prime movers, resulting in shorter circuits that are repeated more times. Please also note that for each example we suggest a loading pattern—low, medium, and high—to ensure progression.

Both load and the total physical demand per circuit must be increased progressively and individually. The example shown in figures 3.5 and 3.6 illustrates that both the load and the training demand pattern increase progressively over time. As the load goes down, the number of repetitions goes up. Please remember that the load changes according to the training demand pattern (refer to the following examples).

For exercises performed against resistance, lower loads are used for entry-level athletes, and slightly heavier loads (and lower reps per set) are used for advanced athletes. Figure 3.6 illustrates an example of a CT combining strength with cardio training (medium-velocity running).

Note to S&C coaches: Please create your own programs based on the needs of the player and equipment available to you.

Exercise	Week 1	2	3	4	5	6
1. Lunges	2 × 15	3 × 12	3 × 10	2 × 10	3 × 8	3 × 6
2. Dumbbell deadlift	2 × 15	3 × 12	3 × 10	2 × 10	3 × 8	3 × 6
3. Bench press	2 × 15	3 × 12	3 × 10	2 × 10	3 × 8	3 × 6
4. Leg curl	2 × 12	3 × 10	3 × 8	2 × 8	3 × 8	3 × 6
5. Upright row	2 × 15	3 × 12	3 × 10	2 × 10	3 × 8	3 × 6
6. Toe raise	2 × 15	3 × 12	3 × 10	2 × 10	3 × 8	3 × 6
7. Running	1× 5 min	1 × 7 min	1 × 10 min	1 × 10 min	1 ×12 min	1 ×15 min

Training-demand pattern

1	2	3	4	5	6
Low	Medium	High	Low	Medium	High

Figure 3.6 Example of a CT program for the A phase for an under-19 player (U19). Cardio can be done between the two circuits, or at the end of the second circuit.

Exercise	Week			Rest interval
	1	2	3	
1. Skipping rope	3 min	2 × 3 min	4 × 2 min	1 min
2. Half squat	2 × 10	3 × 8	3 × 6	2 min
3. Bench press	2 × 10	3 × 8	3 × 6	2 min
4. Front lats pull-down	2 × 10	3 × 8	3 × 6	2 min
5. Toe raise	2 × 15	3 × 12	3 × 10	1 min
6. Ab crunch	2 × 15	3 × 20	3 × 30	1 min
7. Medicine ball (4 kg) chest throw	2 × 8	3 × 8	3 × 10	1 min
8. Low-impact plyometrics	2 × 10	3 × 10	3 × 12	1 min
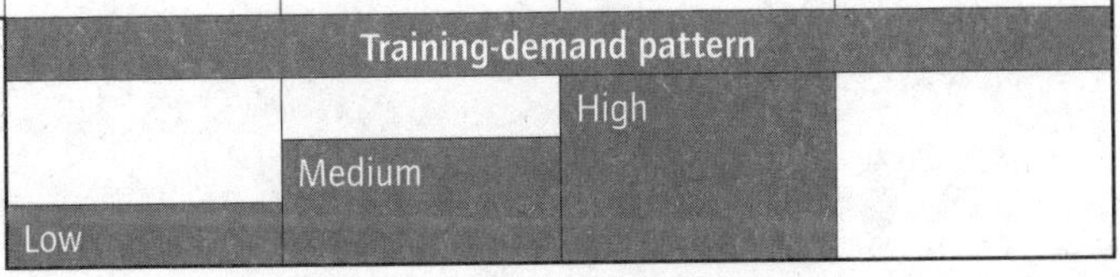 Training-demand pattern				
			High	
		Medium		
Low				

Figure 3.7 An example of a shorter CT plan for a short preparatory phase for U21–23. Skipping rope contributes to cardiorespiratory training.

Cardio training for the adaptation phase can also be of two kinds:

1. Normal running used for distance running. This type of cardio can be used for players who have a longer preparatory phase (6 weeks or longer), such as younger or lower league players, before the official games start, and
2. Tempo running for players from higher leagues, whose time between the end of the league to the beginning of the next one is shorter.

Tempo running is a type of relaxed and upright-position running, over distances between 50–200 m, repeated several times and performed with a speed of approximately 50–75% of maximum: lower speed for the 200 m and 75% for 50–80 m. Please note that as the distance shortens the velocity increases to ready players for the game-specific type of running.

Week 1	Week 2	Week 3	Week 4
10–12 x 200 m	8 x 150 m	8 x 80–100 m	8–10 x 50 m
Intensity: 50%	Intensity: 50–60%	Intensity: 60–70%	Intensity: 70–80%
Rest interval (RI): 2 minutes	RI: 2–3 minutes	RI: 3 minutes	RI: 3–4 minutes

Figure 3.8 A four-week plan for tempo running. The difficulty of the program can be increased or decreased, depending on players' potential and background.

This transition will take the players from the first weeks of adaptation training to the specifics of MxS. As shown in figure 3.9, during the last two weeks (microcycles 5 and 6) of the A phase you can progressively increase training load to 50%, and then to 60% of 1RM so that by the time you start the MxS training your athlete will be ready to use loads of 70% and higher.

Weeks	1	2	3	4	5	6
Training methods	CT using OBW, MB, strength machines, etc.	→	→	→	Strength training: 50-60% 1 RM MB	Strength training: 60-70% 1RM MB

Legend: OBW=own body weight; MB=medicine balls; → = same type of training as in the previous week; 1RM=one repetition maximum

Figure 3.9 Proposed transition of training from CT to MxS.

The adaptation phase of strength training is very important to all players, but specifically for entry-level and beginning individuals. Now is the time when coaches assess players' level of training and, based on that, program future strength training to build a strong foundation for the players. This foundation also represents the time when the coach not only works on strengthening the muscles but most importantly, on fortifying the ligaments and tendons to produce an injury-free player.

Exercise Prescription for the A Phase

The selection of exercises for the adaptation phase is relatively simple. Some of them are presented in figures 3.4–3.7 for many others you can use the equipment available in your gym. However, starting with the A phase and continuing with the other training phases, we will make an analysis of selected exercise used in soccer, suggesting some and being judgmental about others. After all, the intent of this book is to suggest to our readers the best training methods, to combine science with methodology, and to justify scientifically (physiologically and biomechanically) the comments we will make regarding exercise prescription and selection. We will be commenting on what works and what does not.

Soccer players, particularly those in the top echelon, are constantly exposed to various stressful activities: physical, psychological, and socially. This is why we suggest careful attention when you plan your training. Among the S&C instructors there are some who believe that the more exercises the better! If you analyze this method, you will notice that the number of repetitions per exercise is quite low! This view is very questionable, without a basis in science or advanced methodology. Physiologically, this approach is inadequate since it does not result in higher adaptation and, as a result, may not lead to noticeable improvement. Physiologically speaking, efficiency for prime movers means fewer exercises but a higher number of repetitions and sets. This is a clear and successful road to increased overall and local neuromuscular adaptation.

In sports training there are thousands of exercises that are used by S&C instructors. Some of these exercises are very effective at targeting the prime movers, the muscles responsible for performing the most important technical actions in soccer, while others are not. Consequently, an exercise must be selected to fulfill two training roles:

1. To best target the prime movers and,
2. To ensure these muscles will be exposed to a specific physiological adaptation that will result in performance improvement.

This analysis, therefore, will offer some brief remarks about exercises and their importance in strength, power, and agility training.

Despite many decades of strength training, there is still a considerable confusion between strength training for sports and weightlifting, between bodybuilding (big muscles but not quick contracting muscles) and fitness training. Therefore, several comments will refer to what works and what represents just a commercial illusion. Most of the remarks are substantiated by scientific studies, research findings of extreme importance for strength training for sports, and information that will keep us away from personal arguments and opinions.

Most training exercises employed in soccer training can be divided into three categories:

1. **Effective exercises that target the prime movers.** These are the most important exercises that assist the coach in targeting the muscles with the highest contribution to improving sprinting speed, agility, and jumping. One of the best exercises to train the prime movers in soccer is the calf press, where the gastrocnemius—the king of sprinting, agility, and jumping—is effectively targeted.
2. **Exercises that address the ancillary muscles.** These play a secondary role in your exercise selection strategy. Seated leg extension is an ancillary exercise. A suggested ratio is three exercises targeting the prime movers for every exercise targeting ancillary muscles.
3. **Ineffective exercises promoted for commercial reasons or based on some viral trend.** Using these exercises in fitness training represents a disservice to most players, who are using energy and time to perform activities with more than questionable physiological benefit. Since some fake exercises and methods seem to be popular in soccer, physiological training, particularly the area of MxS, speed, speed endurance (lactic acid), and aerobic endurance is inadequate, and players have become prone to injuries.

The methodology of strength training used in soccer must also be scrutinized since it does not meet the needs of being specific to soccer. Since fake training is far from being physiologically demanding, players' readiness for difficult games is often lacking.

The key to training efficiency is the number of repetitions and sets per exercise and not the exercise per se. Why? Because higher repetitions and sets result in higher physiological adaptation of the neuromuscular system. This is the best methodology that results in performance improvements.

Please also remember: the reason for lowering the number of exercises is also based on a key physiological principle: irradiation (Enoka, 2015).

When you perform an exercise, for example a knee extension, the quadriceps muscles are stimulated to contract and perform the action. However, this stimulation does not activate just the rectus femoris, a knee extensor muscle, but also the other muscles surrounding the knee joint. Therefore, you do not need to do other exercises to contract the vastus lateralis and popliteus muscles. Thanks to irradiation these muscles are activated, contracted, and strengthened. Irradiation also helps you to save time and energy and be more efficient in your training.

Always remember this scientific adage: only superior adaptation can result in the highest performance improvement, not useless and ineffective exercises and training methodology.

If there is a secret in sports training, it is specific physiological adaptation. Use this secret to achieve your players' best performance.

You can never display a higher physical potential during the game than the one you have been exposed to during training. Only good training results in high adaptation, and, conversely, to high performance capabilities.

Conclusion

The adaptation (A) phase is essential, not only to build the base of the neuromuscular system but to also use it for injury-prevention programs. Since the A phase is less stressful than the MxS phase, now you can concentrate on

- increasing the flexibility of ankles, knees, and hips and
- strengthening the muscles, ligaments, and tendons of the foot, ankle, knees, and hips.

Do not concentrate only on fitness training with the ball. On the contrary, strength training is more effective when you use strength-training machines. Always remember the unpleasant experience that injuries bring to your sporting life.

Injury prevention should mean stronger muscles, ligaments, and tendons, capable of withstanding the mechanical stress encountered during training and games.

CHAPTER 4
DEVELOPING MAXIMUM STRENGTH TO PRODUCE FAST AND AGILE PLAYERS

KEY POINTS

- The Maximum Strength (MxS) Phase
- The Methodology of Training Maximum Strength
- The Maximum Load Method: The Source of Speed and Agility
- Program Design
- Stiffness and Its Importance in Power, Speed, and Agility
- Exercise Selection for Soccer
- Ineffective Exercises Used in Soccer
- Selected Discussion of Some Training Exercises

Among soccer trainers and players MxS is often grossly misunderstood, evoking images of huge muscles and large, slow players. However, MxS is completely different from what some may imagine. In fact, MxS refers only to the force exerted by a group of muscles or a limb, so it is necessary for improving maximum sprinting speed and agility. Maximum speed and agility are possible only when the prime movers are strong and can apply high force against the ground to project players' body forward as quickly as possible.

The discussion we had in chapter 3 was the prelude to exploring what maximum strength (MxS) is, and what its role is in developing high-quality players. Consequently, **MxS should be considered as the main ingredient to take sprinting speed and agility to the highest level possible**. This is possible because MxS has the physiological capacity to increase the recruitment of fast-twitch muscle fibers resulting in an increased ability of the muscles to contract with higher force and, consequently, produce fast and more agile players.

So do not assume that MxS is not essential in soccer! And do not worry that MxS will make your players big and heavy! This is not the case.

MxS refers only to your own capacity to apply the highest force you can against resistance. Your physique will be as before you trained MxS. You will notice that our suggested training programs tend to focus on your legs, the limbs that generate sprinting speed and agility. This is why in chapters 2 and 3 we explained and justified the role of MxS in the theory of muscle contraction, particularly in the sliding filament theory that initiates and performs muscle contraction.

Note: Without powerful muscle contraction there cannot be fast and agile players.

The Maximum Strength (MxS) Phase

MxS is the mother of all strength-related activities (Schmidtbleicher, 2019).

Professional players need to significantly increase their strength to improve running-based actions, sprinting speed, and agility (Silva et al, 2015)

To be effective for soccer MxS has to be soccer specific, strengthening the prime movers, the muscle groups from the calf, knees, and hips (specifically the gastrocnemius and soleus muscles). The stronger and more powerful the legs, the faster and more reactive and agile the players are. This is why the coach must understand and accept the physiology behind the need to increase MxS. This is the reason we have explained the physiology of muscle contraction, particularly the sliding filament theory. MxS increases the thickness of myosin and the number of cross bridges, and as a result, it will increase the leg's force application against the ground. When a player can apply higher force against the ground during the push-off phase of the running step, they will be faster and more agile.

Consider:

1. If you do not train to increase your MxS, where does your power, speed, and agility come from?
2. To become powerful and fast, some athletes use performance-enhancing substances which may or may not be legal. Rather, performance improvement resulting from increased MxS is superior, natural, and healthy (chapter 2).

The following chapters examine all the necessary information regarding strength training for soccer, and the specific methodology to make your players faster and better.

Training MxS

In soccer we have the soccer field and the player. The field is inert, while the player is the actor, the person moving in various directions throughout the game. Any time the player desires to move in a given direction they apply force against the ground. **The higher the force the player applies against the ground, the higher the sprinting speed they can generate.**

If a forward wants to pass a defender, they have to quickly apply high force against the ground. However, what happens if the attacker does not have the necessary force, and, as such, cannot pass the defender to attempt to score? The only thing the striker can do is to commit to using strength training to increase their legs' force, particularly the MxS of gastrocnemius and soleus. The following information will help you focus on strength training, and better plan your strength training for the future.

Throughout the MxS phase the suggested training load is expressed as a percentage of one repetition maximum (1RM). For this reason, before the beginning of the MxS phase, coaches must test the 1RM for the main exercises, such as calf press and leg press. The 1RM test serves two purposes:

1. to assess the maximum level of your players' strength, and
2. to calculate the load used in training throughout the MxS phase.

Note: We use the term MxS because it refers to the highest load a player can lift. Do not confuse MxS with the bodybuilding method, where the goal of training is big muscles. Strength training for soccer has one major role: to produce fast and agile players.

The Heavy Load Method: The Source of High Speed and Agility

The most effective way to develop MxS is the maximum load method since there is a direct relationship between load and the number of fast-twitch (FT) muscle fibers recruited in action. The heavier the load, the higher the number of muscle fibers recruited in action while performing soccer skills like sprinting and agility moves. The load-muscle recruitment coupling is best expressed by figure 4.1.

As illustrated by figure 4.1a, a lower load, in this example 40% of 1RM, also results in a corresponding lower recruitment of the number of FT fibers (small white circles). For instance, if a soccer player is using a load of 40% during sprinting, his speed will also be lower, proportional to the percentage of FT fibers contracted. One simply cannot generate high sprinting without using a higher number of FT muscle fibers. If, on the other hand, a player recruits in action 60% of his FT muscle fibers (higher number of white circles as compared to the black spots, example 4.1b) his sprinting and agility capabilities are proportionately higher.

Finally, to achieve maximum speed and agility actions a player has to also recruit in action a corresponding higher number of FT fibers. In this case >80–95%. Figure 4.1c exemplifies this reality, where the difference between white and black spots is very visible.

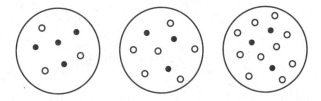

Figure 4.1 The relationship between training loads and the rate of recruitment of fast-twitch muscles fibers.

The scope of MxS is to increase the recruitment of FT muscle fibers in any skill or physical action requiring high speed and agility.

When a player is adapted to the MxS methodology, there will also be a positive transfer to their ability to recruit a high number of FT fibers. As a result, the player will be able to generate high sprinting speed and abrupt agility.

Leg power, so essential in soccer, does not increase by using exercises proposed by commercialism. On the contrary, the ability to run very fast, jump very high, and generate abrupt agility moves are the direct result of applying MxS, power, and agility training methodology.

The use of MxS has the following benefits:

- MxS has a determinant factor in increasing power, maximum speed, and agility.
- It enables the player to reach a high neural output, which is essential for the improvement of power, speed, and agility.
- Along with power training, MxS is part of **central nervous system (CNS) training** (Dorn et al, 2012; Enoka, 2015; Schmidtbleicher, 2019; Duchateau et al, 2021) that increases the firing rate (the frequency of contraction of the fast-twitch muscle fibers) and the discharge rate (the frequency of brain signals sent to the working muscle to contract).
- Therefore, if you do not use MxS during training, do not expect the body to increase the recruitment capacity of fast-twitch muscle fibers, and, as a result, to improve power, speed, and agility.
- Maximum strength is essential for the development of speed and agility not only because it increases the capacity to recruit a high number of muscle fibers, but also since it can apply a higher force against the ground to produce quickness and high velocity.

The loads used for maximum strength development, 70–95% of 1RM, for only one to five reps, result in sets of short duration and, combined with complete rest intervals, allow for the complete restoration of energy (ATP). The MxS load methods also increase testosterone levels, which further explains the improved maximum strength. The level of testosterone in the blood appears to depend on the number and frequency of training sessions per week using the maximum load method (Bangsbo, 2014; Schmidtbleicher, 2019). Testosterone is a male sex hormone that increases muscle mass and muscle strength.

Important elements of success for MxS training with the maximum load method include load, rest interval, exercise order, the speed performing the contraction, and the loading pattern. Maximum strength is developed by increasing the highest possible tension, and, more importantly, by recruiting the highest number of fast-twitch muscle fibers during an athletic action.

Remember that:

* low loads engage slow-twitch muscle fibers and
* loads of greater than 80% of 1RM, moved dynamically, recruit higher numbers of fast-twitch fibers. More importantly, high loads and eccentric methods are even better to increase the thickness of myosin and the number of cross bridges.

Using high loads with few repetitions results in a significant CNS adaptation, better coordination of the muscles involved in a kinetic chain, and an increased capacity to recruit fast-twitch fibers. This is the reason MxS is so important in high-performance soccer; it increases power, speed, and agility. If you do not train MxS, do not expect to improve your players' power, speed, and agility.

The loads used in training also dictate the number of repetitions, sets, and rest intervals planned by a player. The higher the load, the lower the number of repetitions and sets. At the same time, heavy loads also need longer rest intervals between sets to ensure relaxation of CNS, and to recover and replenish energy stores (table 4.1).

Table 4.1 Suggested number of reps per exercise for a training session for MxS

Percent of 1RM	Reps per set	Sets per session	Rest interval between sets/ minutes
70	5–8	5	2-3
75	3–5	4	2-3
80-85	2–3	3	3-4
90	1–2	2	4
95	1	1	4

Rest interval

As part of any training program, rest intervals (RI) between sets are based on the type of training and the players' fitness potential and should be calculated to ensure adequate recovery of the neuromuscular system. For loads of 70–80% of 1RM, a RI of 2–3 minutes between sets is sufficient for both CNS and ATP-CP recovery. For the maximum load method of 80–90 % 1RM, a RI of 3–5 minutes is necessary because maximum loads heavily tax the CNS, which therefore takes longer to recover. If the RI is much shorter, CNS participation could plummet in terms of maximum concentration, motivation, and the power of nerve impulses sent to the contracting muscles (Robinson et al, 1995; Lephart and Karunakara, 1997; Pincivero and Campy, 2004; Pandy, 2021). Insufficient rest may also jeopardize complete restoration of the required energy fuel for contraction (ATP-CP).

When discussing rest intervals, we should also consider other aspects of sports training, such as the stress players are exposed to and exercises which are not beneficial for increasing strength. Players are constantly taxed by various stressors, from physical to social, from intellectual activities to family stress.

Beware of players' resting, recovery, and regeneration activities, and constantly improve them. Remember, a well-rested player can train more efficiently and be ready for the games to follow.

> High intensity (load) with long rest intervals is the best method to improve MxS because it increases muscle activation and the recruitment of fast-twitch muscle fibers.

Speed of Contraction

During any strength-training program players use a variety of loads. The implemented loads dictate the speed of contraction, or how quick a strength-training action is performed. Many soccer actions are often performed quickly, dynamically. This is why players should perform fast, dynamic contractions from the middle of the preparatory phase throughout the league games. As a result of quick actions, the neuromuscular system will adapt to quickly recruit fast-twitch muscle fibers, while the players' application of force against resistance (the ground and gravity) must be exerted as dynamically as possible.

The desire to quickly apply force in the shortest amount of time is fundamental for the positive transfer of the neuromuscular adaptations to the specific needs of soccer. High motivation and maximum concentration are fundamental qualities necessary for the activation of MxS and power. Only a high speed of contraction performed against a high load will quickly recruit fast-twitch fibers, resulting in the highest increase in maximum strength, power, speed, and agility (González-Badillo et al, 2014; Schmidtbleicher, 2019; Pandy, 2021).

S&C trainers and coaches should note that in the case of maximum loads, such as 90% 1RM, the speed of contraction looks slow and moves slow, but the application of force against resistance has to be fast in order to recruit the highest number of fast-twitch muscle fibers necessary to overcome resistance.

Program Design

Since soccer has many dynamic actions that place a high demand on the neuromuscular system, most players can perform MxS two times a week. To train MxS three times per week is suggested only for elite players with a stronger training background. Do not, however, be alarmed at the difficulty of this program. On the contrary, the MxS program suggested in table 4.2. can be followed by all soccer players from top leagues because the most difficult element in MxS is not the number of repetitions but rather the number of sets. Or, in our example (table 4.2) the players do not exceed four sets. During the league games, this can be reduced to one to two maximum load sessions per week, often performed in combination with other strength components, such as power.

Table 4.2 An example of a three-microcycle (weeks) training for a player that has a short time to focus on MxS

Exercise/ Microcycle	1	2	3	Rest interval
Leg press	75/6/3	80/3/4	85/3/4	3-4
Front lats pull-down	70/6/3	80/4/4	85/3-4/4	3-4
Calf press	80/6/3	85/4/4	85/3-4/4	3-4

Notation program: Example from top left cell: 75=75% of 1RM; 3 =number of reps; 3 =number of sets

Please adapt the program suggested in table 4.2 to the player. Do not be surprised if some players can do a more challenging program, such as higher load and sets, particularly for leg exercises.

The notation of load, number of reps, and number of sets can also be expressed as follows: under week 1 in table 4.3, the numerator (e.g., 70) refers to the load as a percentage of 1RM, the denominator (e.g., 3) represents the number of reps, and the multiplier (e.g., 3) indicates the number of sets. During each of the lower steps, a 1RM testing session is planned for the latter part of the week, when the player has better recovered from the strain of the preceding high step.

Table 4.3 Sample MxS for a soccer team (lower leagues and U19 players) where the preparatory phase is longer

Exercise	Rest interval	Week					
		1	2	3	4	5	6
Leg press	3	$\frac{70}{3} \times 3$	$\frac{75}{4} \times 3$	$\frac{80}{5\text{-}6} \times 4$	$\frac{75}{3} \times 3$	$\frac{80}{5} \times 4$	$\frac{85}{3} \times 4$
Bench press	3-4	$\frac{70}{3} \times 4$	$\frac{80}{3} \times 3$	$\frac{70}{1} \times 4$	$\frac{80}{3} \times 3$	$\frac{85}{3} \times 3$	$\frac{85}{3} \times 4$
Front lat pulldown	2	$\frac{75}{3} \times 3$	$\frac{80}{3} \times 3$	$\frac{80}{3} \times 3$	$\frac{80}{3} \times 3$	$\frac{85}{4} \times 3$	$\frac{85}{3} \times 3$
Leg curl	2-3	2 x 8	3 x 8	3 x 10	2 x 8	3 x 8	3 x 10
Calf press	3	$\frac{80}{5} \times 3$	$\frac{85}{4} \times 4$	$\frac{85}{3} \times 3$	$\frac{80}{4} \times 4$	$\frac{85}{4} \times 4$	$\frac{90}{3} \times 3$
Training demand pattern		Low	Medium	High	Low	Medium	High

Note: Leg press and calf press are the essential prime movers for sprinting, while the bench press may be replaced with another exercise.

Another example of MxS is illustrated by table 4.4, a program suitable for players that plan a shorter MxS phase. Since the load increases, from 70-85%, relatively quickly, we suggest this program for players with a good strength-training background. Please also note that such a program does not take too much time. Yet, at the end of it, you will notice clear improvements. However, if you can dedicate the time for another cycle of three weeks your players will be better athletes. If your players cannot spare much time and energy, you can decrease the overall physiological stress by reducing the number of sets to just two.

Table 4.4 A hypothetical example of a three-week MxS for elite players with a shorter MxS phase but a better background in strength training.

Exercises	Week 1	Week 2	Weeks 3	Rest interval
Leg press	$\frac{70 \times 3}{6}$	$\frac{80 \times 4}{6}$	$\frac{85 \times 4}{5}$	3
Leg curls	$\frac{70 \times 3}{6}$	$\frac{75 \times 4}{8}$	$\frac{80 \times 3}{5}$	4
Calf press	$\frac{80 \times 4}{7}$	$\frac{85 \times 4}{8}$	$\frac{85 \times 4}{4}$	3

By now, the needs and benefits of MxS training should be clear since stronger players will become more powerful, faster, and more agile. Improvements of MxS will help players apply higher force against the ground (push-off phase of the running step), improve speed, improve reactivity, and discourage aggressive opponents.

Stiffness and Its Importance in Power, Speed, and Agility

Stiffness refers to the capacity of the kinetic chain of the body (ankle, knees, hips, the low back, and spinal column) to resist deformation and to not collapse on ground contact during sprinting, jumping, and agility actions. Vertical stiffness can be best described as a leg spring or could be an analogous with a bouncing ball.

Imagine you hold in your hands two balls: one made from stiff rubber and, the other one, a typical, soft beach ball. You release both at the same time. When the soft ball lands, because of its soft material, it deforms and absorbs elastic energy. As a result, it rebounds at lower height. The stiffer ball, on the other hand, resists deformation, while the stored elastic energy makes the ball rebound higher.

The same occurrence is visible in soccer, mostly in sprinting, jumps, and agility actions. Loose ankles, muscles, ligaments, and tendons affect the players' capacity to absorb the impact of landing. The stronger the muscles and tendons (particularly the Achilles tendon), the faster and more agile a player is. Maximum strength (MxS) has a substantial contribution to stiffness by strengthening players' muscles, ligaments, and tendons. However, if a player's MxS is modest, maximum stiffness is clearly affected, and, as a result, so is maximum speed, jump power, and agility. This impediment is visible when you test the duration of the leg's contact phase on the ground. A shorter contact phase means stronger legs and vertical stiffness which manifests in a stronger rebound during powerful types of athletic actions.

Selected Comments Regarding Stiffness

- The highest vertical stiffness is reached during maximum speed and various jumps as a reflection of good neural and muscle reactivity.
- Strong muscles might also be slow because of the slower speed of the sliding filaments and the speed of the overlapping of myosins with actins. **MxS is the only option to overcome that since heavy loads can recruit a higher number of fast-twitch muscle fibers and can increase the myosin thickness. The obvious result is an increase in the quickness of contraction, translated into faster and more agile players.**
- Elite sprinters have a shorter duration of contact phase and vertical stiffness (Nagahara et al, 2017; Del Vechio et al, 2021; Duchateau et al, 2021; Villamar et al, 2021).
- **Stiffness increases proportionately with the weight on the ankle** during strength training (Matos et al, 2021).
- The same authors claim that men have greater stiffness than women. This can be corrected by using MxS methodology to improve MxS.
- Strong stiffness is determinant for fast sprinting, reactive actions, agility, and reactive jumps, and it is directly dependent on the force of the gastrocnemius and soleus.

- Ankle stiffness increases only when maximum strength (MxS) is increased. There is strong interdependence between the two factors for the benefit of those who want to be fast and agile.
- Strong muscles are very important in athletics, but stiff tendons, the Achilles tendon in particular, are the secret weapon for high speed, power, and agility. Lower stiffness of the Achilles tendon results in lower speed.
- Muscles are remarkably strong: the weight of the calf muscles is just a kilogram, but they can lift 500 kg (Blazevich, 2021).
- The development of maximum speed depends on muscle power as well as on ankle joint stiffness (Nagahara and Zushi, 2017).
- Enoka (2015) claims that the Achilles tendon has the strongest stiffness of all muscles: 2,857 N/cm or 291 kg/cm, or 641.5 Lbs. Strong stiffness is determinant for fast sprinting, reactive actions, agility, and reactive jumps, and it is directly dependent on the force of gastrocnemius and soleus.

Stiffness and Injuries

- **Ankle sprains** are among the most common injuries, often resulting from ankle instability and inadequate strengthening of the joints forming the kinetic chains.
- Of those with ankle sprains, 30–40% also develop **ankle instability** (Matos et al, 2021).
- Charalambous and colleagues (2011) identified that **joint stiffness is an important performance-related variable**, and a positive power producer. However, these authors have also cautioned that **low stiffness can be associated with injuries**.
- **Injury prevention means stronger muscles, ligaments, tendons, and stiffness**, capable of withstanding the mechanical stress encountered during training and competitions.

Exercise Selection for Strength Training: A Brief Professional Analysis

The world of exercise selection for soccer is still an unsettled debate with too many suggestions of exercises coming from people with a questionable understanding of sports science and training methodology.

- Our analysis is made from the position of former top and international class athletes and coaches. Prior to sharing information with you, we have also been in the trenches of top athletic competitions.
- This analysis is not based on opinions, but rather on the results of research studies. Research results and conclusions drawn from a study are based on scientific testing, on comparing one theory to another. As a result, we will share with you what is effective in training and what is not.
- The internet is a wilderness, but an important one for our freedom, where everybody can suggest anything they want and propose unproven theories and exercises.
- Before making any decisions about exercise selection, please read the information we share with you regarding the suggested training programs for the A and MxS phases.
- For our analysis of exercises proposed by commercialism we have selected just a low number. It is up to you to extend your judgment from this analysis to other exercises: Are they effective? Or not?
- Commercialized exercise programs offer gadgets to perform some exercises, most of which are not efficient, with the weight of the implement being far too low (3–5 kg) to have an impact on the development of MxS and power. As already mentioned, low loads do not elicit the recruitment of fast-twitch muscle fibers and, as a result, do not improve strength, power, and agility.
- If you analyze some of the trending exercises, you might, as we did, draw the conclusion that the proponents of these exercises have good intentions but a very diluted knowledge of sports training.

In the tradition of strength training for soccer, heavy loads are rarely used. Just because a player can lift a dumbbell of 5 kg, it should not give you the illusion that this is an exercise for strength or that it will improve strength. Despite the dominant role maximum strength (MxS) has in speed-power sports, in generating rapid actions, and in maximum speed and quick changes of direction, this type of strength training is quite uncommon in soccer.

- **Question 1:** If training for the development of MxS is not common, what type of activity do you do to improve power, speed, and agility?
- **Question 2:** Why do so many of the currently popular exercise programs require you to use a gadget or training accessory?
- **Question 3:** What is important in soccer training: selecting an exercise based on current fads, or choosing training programs based on the physiology of soccer?

The pressure placed by current commercial fitness trends on soccer clubs and players (including on athletes from other sports) to use ineffective exercises and gear is quite high. Please consider the following discussion about selected exercises and draw your own conclusion.

Stability Ball

Stability ball exercises seem to be quite popular among some soccer clubs and coaches. Exercises done on this ball are purported to develop strength and improve balance. Although research on balance training has not reached a scientific verdict yet, there are many studies that claim there is no proof that balance training develops strength, or that it results in any sort of athletic benefit (Fisher et al, 2011; Benis et al, 2016; Schedler et al, 2020). It might develop proprioception, the sense of body awareness while exercising, but that will not help a player to develop speed and agility.

Battle Rope

Using a battle rope, or fitness rope, is good exercise for overall fitness. It increases overall strength and cardio for the average fitness enthusiast. The muscles activated in this exercise are the legs, mostly contracted isometrically; shoulder muscles; and the back (intervertebral and lumbar muscles). The low back muscles are activated mostly isometrically, as a support for the trunk and hips throughout the duration of the exercise.

Strength training for soccer requires specificity, or exercises that address the prime movers. Therefore, if you want to use this exercise for your players, do it during the early part of the annual plan (A phase). After that, particularly during the MxS training, exercises must be very specific, along the direction of muscle contraction and must address the prime movers for soccer.

Elastic Resistance Bands

Elastic cords were first used in Romania in rowing (1954) to develop muscle endurance with lower resistance pulls performed up to 250 repetitions non-stop (the approximate number of strokes used during a race). Since the late 1970s elastic cords have become very popular among fitness enthusiasts. Elastic cords and bands are quite effective for general fitness training but are ineffective for sports where power is an important physical attribute.

Consider that the force against the starting blocks applied by a top sprinter is 174 kg for the rear leg and 168 kg for the front leg, whereas a band's resistance is around 20-60 kg, and often the higher resistance bands are not used in fitness training for soccer players (Francis and Bompa, personal notes).

It seems, then, that resistance bands are not effective when it comes to training soccer players' leg power. In addition, their resistance increases as you stretch them, which is exactly opposite to what happens in power actions, sprinting, and agility moves, where resistance is higher at the beginning of the push-off. Maximum force and quick leg action occurs towards the end of a running step (such as the push-off/propulsion phase of the running step). Therefore, when you use an elastic band, its resistance is highest at the end of the stretch, inhibiting acceleration and quickness of action.

Effective Training Exercises for Soccer

If S&C coaches are still unsure about the most effective type of strength training and strength-training techniques that will best serve their players, the following discussion should shed some light on what is effective for soccer players, and what is not:

- Always remember that skills and athletic motions are made by muscles. Muscles always behave as per the training program you expose them to. If you expose muscles to heavy loads, they adapt to that, resulting in fast running, high jumping, and abrupt agility actions during the game. If you use ineffective exercises for 4-8 seconds, the standard soccer program proposed by commercialism, your players will have a hard time completing a game with high intensity.

- For the best physiological benefit, **exercises employed during training must be performed along the same neural pathway used during sprinting, jumping**, and kicking the ball (Hakkinen, 1989; Schmidtbleicher, 2019; Pandy et al, 2021; Matos et al, 2022). This means that to be soccer-specific, exercises must be selected so that the muscles' contractions during the exercise are performed in the same direction, angle, posture, and sequence occurs during sprinting, jumping, and agility actions. If prime movers are not realistically stimulated, not specific, the result will be lower exercise transfer and low specific improvement.

- Motor unit recruitment and firing rate increase when training loads are higher and muscle contractions are faster (De Luca et al, 1982; Kunugi et al, 2021). Training methods that enhance maximum strength and power are the only ones that increase fast-twitch muscle fiber recruitment and the firing rate of motor units (Schmidtbleicher, 2019; Duchateau et al, 2021). If these physiological actions do not occur, you will likely be unsuccessful in improving your players' power, speed, and agility.

- If you follow this essential physiological concept, you must reject the vast majority of gadgets that are promoted online as they lack scientific backing as to their effectiveness.

Comparing Strength-Training Exercises: A Scientific Justification

Squats vs Leg and Calf Press

Since legs are the essential limbs in soccer, we will analyze some exercises that will have important benefits for soccer players in their quest to become faster and more agile.

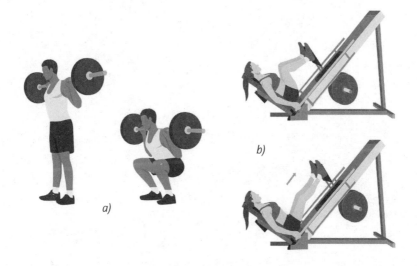

Figure 4.2 (a) A traditional barbell squat exercise. (b) A calf press exercise that targets gastrocnemius muscle, an important muscle for running and agility.

Many instructors still believe squats and deep squats are the most effective exercises for the legs (calf and knees extensor muscles), but several research studies in exercise physiology and biomechanics demonstrate that during active squats, vastus lateralis has a higher contribution than rectus femoris.

Furthermore, during a squat exercise, soleus and gastrocnemius, the determinant muscles during sprinting, jumping, and agility, have a low to minimal contribution (Escamilla, 2001; Robertson et al, 2008; Dorn et al, 2012; Morin et al, 2015; Monte et al, 2020; Pandy et al, 2021). In other words, squats have mostly a vertical, upward, impulse but little benefit to the push-off in speed and agility training. Suggestion: Replace squats with leg and calf presses (figure 4.2b) or calf raises (figure 4.3).

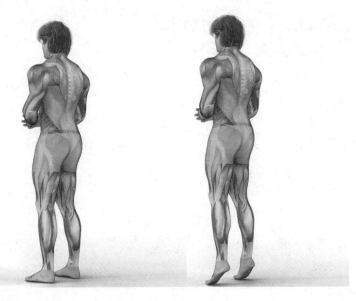

Figure 4.3 An example of calf raises. Please note the range of ankle plantar and dorsiflexion, very essential for the maximization of gastrocnemius and soleus muscles.

The muscle most activated during squats are quadriceps (vastus lateralis and rectus femoris) and to some extent, the hamstrings, glutes, and lumbar muscles. As concluded by the above researchers, squats have a minimal contribution to strengthening gastrocnemius and soleus.

During squats, gastrocnemius is mostly activated as a stabilizer, not as a prime mover, lifter, or producer of force. Instead, you should perform leg presses, particularly calf raises and calf presses, the most effective exercises to target and train gastrocnemius and soleus.

Finally, soccer professionals concerned about knee and calf injuries should know that calf and leg presses have the lowest risk of injury whereas squats have the highest. Equally important is that squats have the lowest activation for gastrocnemius and soleus, the determinant muscles in sprinting and agility.

Unilateral Squats and Other Unilateral Leg Exercises

Some strength-training instructors prefer unilateral (one leg) to bilateral (two legs) squats in the belief that the former is a more effective exercise. The reality, however, is exactly the opposite. Elliasen et al (2018) have conducted a comparison study of unilateral vs bilateral squats. Their conclusion was that during the bilateral squat, muscle activation was significantly greater, particularly rectus femoris, compared to unilateral squats. During bilateral squats, a player's stability is better, and the soccer player can lift superior weight that translates into recruiting a higher number of muscle fibers (McCurdy et al, 2004; Khuu et al, 2016; Bompa and Sarandan, 2023).

Unilateral squats, however, are necessary only under one condition: to balance the eventual discrepancy between the strength potential of the two legs. Consequently, unilateral squats and exercises are less effective for athletes and, to some degree, a waste of time and energy.

Some coaches and instructors are visibly reluctant about strength training, believing that strength might increase muscle mass and, as a result, increase players' body weight. There is, however, a strength-training methodology that allows them to increase strength capabilities without increasing muscle mass: nervous system training (Schmidtbleicher, 1984; Enoka, 1988 and 2015; Zatsiorski, 1995; Seitz et al, 2014; Bompa and Buzzichelli, 2019). This specific strength training is also part of the entire training system we propose in this book. However, a variant of this methodology calls for lower loads performed faster (power training), which is advisable mostly for teams that have a shorter preparatory phase. In addition, it is the best training for the improvement of power, speed, and agility without increasing muscle mass or players' weight.

Jump Squats

Jump squat is a very effective exercise for developing leg power (quadriceps, gastrocnemius, and soleus muscles), mostly during the propulsion phase of the jump. Start the upwards action with the thighs in a horizontal position, and progressively accelerate upward ending in a vertical jump and forward medicine ball throw.

As you begin to initiate the vertical jump and perform a take-off, the gastrocnemius becomes an effective producer of force via its push-off against the ground.

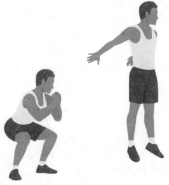

Figure 4.4. The jump squat.

Deadlifts

Traditionally, a deadlift is used to strengthen the leg (including calf and quadriceps), buttocks (gluteus), and low-back muscles (lumbar and intervertebral).

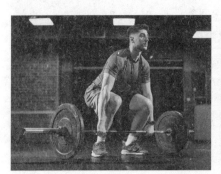 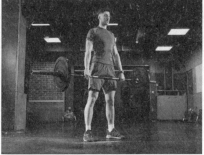

Figure 4.5 The deadlift.

However, an electromyography (EMG) analysis by Martin-Fuentes (2020) revealed that calf muscles do not have even a minimal activation during deadlifts. Therefore, if your goal is to strength the calf muscles, it is better to do calf presses rather than deadlifts.

Deadlifts, particularly the Romanian deadlift variant, do address the hamstrings, biceps femoris, and glutes, but can also strengthen the lumbar and intervertebral muscles. A careful load, and good technique, is beneficial also to the development of the trunk in general, improving its supporting, stability, and capacity during many actions performed by legs and arms. A good progression regarding the load is a simplified technique, where you reduce the angles of knee and hip flexion.

TRX Frame for Group Training

Training equipment companies are constantly offering novel fitness-training options, including the TRX frame. The TRX frame is specifically used for suspension exercises intended to train arm strength, through pulling and pushing. However, this type of strength training for the arms has little benefit in the overall training program of the soccer player.

Conclusions

Chapter 4 discussed MxS and the methods necessary to develop it. The most important conclusion to draw from this discussion is the positive effect of MxS on the development of soccer-specific abilities, such as power, sprinting speed, agility, and reactivity.

Though, with many clubs all over the world, MxS is not a very popular training concept. There are still some soccer professionals who question the needs of MxS in soccer. To them, strength equals big muscles!

Let us repeat the question once more: if you do not train MxS, particularly for the propulsion muscles (gastrocnemius and soleus), where is the power necessary to generate fast speed and agility coming from? What do you use to improve the force necessary to produce a fast player?

We suggest that if you instead apply the methods we propose for the development of MxS, gains in the size of gastrocnemius will be minimal. However, the improvement of MxS and, as a result, the increase in maximum sprinting capabilities from the improvement of MxS will be categorically visible.

Soccer players are pressed for time, and spending hours on ineffective and non-sport-specific exercises can be a waste of valuable time and energy without any benefit. Too much time is often spent on ineffective, very short agility drills in soccer and not enough on MxS, power, and specific endurance that help to improve soccer-specific qualities.

Coaches and instructors should review their training philosophy by creating a neuromuscular strategy to improve effectiveness.

A final suggestion: Simplify your training and reduce the number of exercises as much as possible. Simple is beautiful. And also saves time and energy.

CHAPTER 5
TESTING AND ASSESSING CONTEMPORARY PHYSICAL TRAINING IN SOCCER

By Sorin O. Sarandan, PhD

For many years soccer training has been constantly exposed to many changes, some based on science and methodology, others originating from some sports equipment companies. The internet, certainly, is another medium of influence, often coming from readily available gurus, enthusiastically sharing their theories of the moment. All these sources share novel training methods for the development of strength, power, speed, agility, and specific endurance. The world of science, research, and science-based methodology, on the other hand, is rarely consulted. This is why some strength and conditioning (S&C) instructors might be confused. Who is right and whose theories should we follow?

Scientific Assessment of Contemporary Physical Training in Soccer

Since contemporary training seems so conflicted, with many theories resulting in undesirable results, we have decided to conduct an investigation to assess the benefits of contemporary training vs. what we promote in this book. Which is best? Which one has a visible impact on the development of physical qualities dominant in team sports? The entire organization and methodology of our investigation is presented next.

Research Hypothesis

That a science-based strength training methodology will result in superior development of team-sports-specific dominant abilities, such as strength, power, maximum speed, and agility.

Subjects and Duration of Experiment

Two groups of 14 boys' U17 soccer players were selected from local youth championships:

- the **experimental group** was formed by the ASU Politehnica Timisoara soccer players, and
- the **reference group** were soccer players from the Sports High School Timisoara team.

Duration of the experiment: A three-month period of S&C training programs beginning in early January 2020 and ending at the end of April of the same year. This period coincided with the preparatory phase for the local championships.

Number of training sessions of S&C per week: Three for both groups

Testing: A standard *test-retest* format was followed by both groups.

Training Programs

The experimental group (ASU Politehnica) followed a periodized strength, power, agility, and maximum speed training as explained in this book:

- **AA (Anatomical Adaptation):** Three weeks
- **MxS for six weeks:** using progressively heavier loads of 50–70% 1RM
- **Power, agility, maximum speed:** Three weeks

The reference group (Sports High School) followed an independent, contemporary training program for soccer organized by the team's trainers:

- Maximum speed runs of 1030 meters
- Agility runs: Slalom and zigzag, agility ladder, agility rings on flat terrain and over low hurdlers of 4–10 seconds
- Resistance trainer: Speed sled
- Circuits of jumps over boxes, pull-ups, push-ups, stepping on Bosu balls
- Medicine balls throws
- Strength training using elastic cords: Pulls and presses for arms and legs

Testing Protocols and Results

Testing procedures are listed below while their results, with comments and conclusions, are at the end of this chapter. All the necessary comments are technical but presented in a brief and simple manner. Conclusions, on the other hand, will be used to demonstrate whether our hypothesis was substantiated or just an imagination.

Testing Players' Power Using Myotest

Myotest is a portable instrument equipped with sensors to detect any movements made by the athletes and measure force and power with a strong positive correlation, $r=0.96$, and a high probability, $p<0.05$ (Comstock et al, 2011; Orange et al, 2019). Myotest also has an accelerometer that measures:

- duration of contact time (duration of players' feet on the ground during maximum speed and take-off to perform a jump)
- reactivity, the proportion of jump's height and duration of contact time
- stiffness, the proportion between the force applied against the ground and the degree of vertical deformation during sprinting and jumping (Poorly trained players with low strength capabilities cannot overcome the force of gravity and react quickly between landing and take-off or during sprinting and repetitive jumps.)

Myotest has been used for testing:

- **Countermovement jumps (CMJ)** are reactive jumps used to assess force, power, height, and speed. Performance in CMJ is directly correlated to sprinting capabilities and 1RM.
- **Jump-plyometric (JP)** can provide information regarding the duration of contact on the ground, the contractile properties of the muscles, reactivity, and muscle stiffness, all of which are essential to improving athleticism and performance in the chosen sport.

Testing Maximum Strength (MxS)

The information regarding MxS for athletes in the form of one repetition maximum (1RM) is essential:

1. to know players' MxS and
2. to calculate the load for the duration of training for MxS. Three tests were used for the major muscles groups used in soccer:

- **Leg press** assesses the 1RM for leg extensors (quadriceps muscles).
- **Calf press** targets the most important muscles in team sports involving running and jumping: gastrocnemius and soleus.
- **Bench press** is mostly trained to block the opponents during the game in the penalty area.

Testing Maximum Speed and Agility

Speed and agility are essential qualities in team sports. This justifies why we need this information to assess players' maximum speed and agility, such as:

- **Maximum speed test:** 30 m sprint from a standing position
- **Agility: Illinois test**, organized on a flat surface (grass or gym) using eight cones to mark the turning points during the test. Players start the test by resting on the back on the floor. At a signal the athlete stands up and runs as fast as possible following the design of the illustrated test. The coach records the time to determine the best performance.

Testing Results and Discussions

All the results from our testing protocol are presented in a table format that allows you to make direct and relevant comparisons between the experimental and reference groups. We were also very selective with different tests, focusing mostly on testing the major abilities specific to team sports. Specific and relevant discussions are also made for each test, their meaning, and their correlation between some tests with the dominant abilities in team sports, such as maximum speed and agility.

Table 5.1 Mean testing results for each group of players for the countermovement jump (CMJ)

	Group	Test	Retest
Height in cm	Experimental	32.71	35.47
	Reference	32.59	33.35
Power: W/kg	Experimental	40.59	45.32
	Reference	43.19	46.68
Force/N	Experimental	23.74	26.43
	Reference	24.75	25.61
Speed of CMJ in cm/s	Experimental	223.41	239.76
	Reference	221.16	231.33

W/kg = Watts per kg; Force/N = force in Newton (unlike the measure of force in kg/lb, the advantage of using N is that it also considers the mass, the weight of the subject)

Comments: Please note that for the first test, there was not a significant difference between the two groups. However, the retest scores revealed a consistent improvement for the experiment group in the *tests for height (3 vs 1 cm), power (5 vs 1.5 W), force (3 vs 1 N), and speed of CMJ (16.35 vs.10.17 cm/s)*

Conclusions: The significant improvement in the power and force tests for the experimental group also explains why height and speed of CMJ were better than for the reference group. For practical purposes, the most important improvement appears to be the speed of CMJ which will allow a player to be more reactive and move faster in various aspects of the game.

Table 5.2 Mean value per group for jump plyometric (JP) test

	Group	Test	Retest
Duration of contact time in mls	Experimental	170.75	174.66
	Reference	159.41	160.75
Stiffness (kn/m)	Experimental	35.18	35.95
	Reference	41.75	39.57
Power (W)	Experimental	31.33	34.54
	Reference	30.40	30.36

mls = milliseconds; kn/m= kilonewton/meter; W = Watts

Comments: Duration of contact time decreased 4.09 mls for the experimental group and 1.34 mls for the reference group. This proves that there is a significant correlation between improvement in leg strength and a decrease in the duration of contact time. In practical terms, this means that these players can run faster, change direction much quicker, and have faster reactions during the dynamic parts of the games.

Conclusions: The results of the jump plyometric test demonstrate that improvement in power directly correlates with a decrease in the duration of contact time. The shorter the duration of contact time, the faster and more reactive and agile the athletes are—qualities any coach wants for their athletes.

Table 5.3 Mean values for the MxS tests

	Group	Test	Retest
Leg press (kg)	Experimental	96.67	129.83
	Reference	76.64	83.33
Calf press (kg)	Experimental	84.00	99.58
	Reference	54.58	59.58
Bench press (kg)	Experimental	58.41	68.75
	Reference	53.33	56.25

Comments: The results of MxS tests demonstrate the highest (high significance) difference between the mean scores of the experimental and reference groups: 26.5 kg. The same difference was visible for the calf press: 10.6 kg. These differences demonstrate that the training program followed by the experimental group has resulted in visible gains in all the tests where strength, power, and jumping abilities have been assessed.

In MxS tests leg press and calf press significantly improved for the experimental group by 33.2 kg for leg press and by 22.7 kg for calf press. At the same time, the improvement of MxS for the reference group was marginal: 6.7 kg for leg press and 2.9 kg for calf press.

Conclusions: Considering the modest improvements recorded for the reference group, it is very difficult to expect to improve the determinant abilities, speed and agility, in soccer and most other team sports.

Do you want to visibly improve your players' strength, power, maximum speed, and agility? Change your S&C training program.

Table 5.4 Results of 30 m maximum speed and Illinois agility test

	Group	Test	Retest
30 m maximum speed (sec)	Experimental	4.74	4.49
	Reference	4.61	4.60
Illinois agility test (sec)	Experimental	16.55	16.14
	Reference	16.36	16.42

Comments: While the scores for the reference group were relatively flat for both tests, the experimental group had an improvement of 0.25 seconds for the 30 m maximum speed and 0.41 seconds for the Illinois agility test. The discrepancy between the two groups demonstrates that the experimental group has improved the speed-agility performance simply because the strength-power scores have improved.

Conclusions

- Gains in strength-power have been translated into improvements in speed-agility.
- The initial tests did not reveal a significant difference for the test scores between the two groups. However, the retest data demonstrated a statistically significant difference for the improvement of strength between the two groups, $p = 0.032 < 0.05$, and a validity of 95%.
- There is clear evidence that our working hypothesis has been proven to be correct and that the test results have demonstrated that the increase of players' strength in the experimental group has resulted in visibly improved maximum speed and agility, the two determinant abilities in team sports.
- There is a strong correlation between improvements in strength-power with the increase of maximum speed-agility.
- You can be fast only if you improve your strength and power first.
- *In practical terms this means that contemporary physical training in soccer is, at best, very modest, with a slow rate of performance improvement.*

This discussion about MxS and its methodology to create a faster and more agile soccer player is of great importance for all soccer professionals, not only for the purpose of learning what MxS is and how to train it, but to also accept a novel training methodology.

We would also like to ask you to review the sliding filament theory in chapter 2 and connect this information with the theoretical concept of training MxS. Now you will be equipped with both theory and practical application.

PART III
TRANSFORMING MAXIMUM STRENGTH INTO SOCCER-SPECIFIC ABILITIES

Part III is the essential section of the book for soccer professionals, coaches, and S&C instructors alike since now we are discussing how to transform gains in MxS into the determinant qualities needed to succeed in soccer.

In chapter 4 we demonstrated the importance of MxS in producing quick, fast, and agile soccer players. Although gains in MxS are important for your players, it cannot be used in its crude form, since soccer is a fast game played for 90 minutes, where the actual abilities, from speed to endurance, are used at a maximum.

Therefore, to benefit from the improvement of MxS, we have to convert it, transform it into soccer-specific abilities such as power, agility, sprinting speed, and endurance. It is our hope that you will examine this text with an open mind. It is not traditional information, since we discuss the needs in soccer from a slightly different position, that of using more strength training, particularly MxS, since this ability is determinant for the development of power, speed, and agility. Your players will be faster and more agile than in the past years.

CHAPTER 6
TRANSFORMING MXS INTO
SOCCER-SPECIFIC POWER

KEY POINTS

- Physiological Strategy to Increase Power
- Program Design for Power Training
- Ballistic Method
- Plyometric Method
- Power Training for Soccer
- Power Endurance
- Starting Power
- Acceleration Power
- Deceleration Power
- Training Goalkeepers

Gains in MxS are essential for the development of soccer-specific abilities, specifically for the development of power. Power training is in fact a transition from MxS to soccer-specific speed and agility, the most sought-after physical qualities for soccer players.

For soccer, a sport where speed-dynamic actions are determinant to achieve the proposed objective for a team, power is an essential ingredient that requires a high rate of force and quickness of action. In sports science power is defined as the rate of producing force (Enoka, 2002, 2015).

In order to improve performance and make your players the most effective, you have to increase power, speed, and physical resilience to overcome fatigue. A player can be very strong, with a large muscle mass, yet be unable to display power because of an inability to contract already strong muscles in a very short time.

The advantage of dynamic power training is that it trains the central nervous system (CNS). Therefore, improvements in performance can be based on neural changes that help individual muscles achieve greater performance capability (Sale, 1986; Roig et al, 2009; Schmidtbleicher, 2019). This gain is accomplished by shortening the time required to recruit motor units especially of fast-twitch fibers (Häkkinen and Komi, 1983; Enoka, 2015; Pandy et al, 2021).

Power-training methodology and exercises employed during this training phase activate and increase the discharge rate and the quickness of contraction of fast-twitch muscle fibers, leading to specific CNS adaptations. This adaptation shows itself in the form of discharging a greater number of muscle fibers in a very short time. Both training practice and research have shown that such adaptations require considerable time and that they progress from year to year.

During the transformation phase from MxS to power, exercises must be performed quickly and dynamically in order to recruit the highest number of F T muscle fibers at the highest rate of contraction. The entire program should be geared toward achieving only one goal: to display force in a dynamic manner, explosively. Coaches should select only those training methods that fulfill the requirements of power development, that is, methods that enhance quickness, facilitate explosive application of force, and increase the reactivity of the relevant muscles.

Physiological Strategy to Increase Power

Although most soccer professionals recognize that the physiology of soccer is very complex, covering the entire range of physical abilities, from speed to endurance, they also admit that training to improve each ability is not very simple. Yet some professionals adhere to a very innocent philosophy: if you want to be fast, you have to train short-distance sprinting; if you want to increase power, you have to do only power drills; and if you want to improve agility, you have to train short agility exercises, such as speed lather drills. What about aerobic endurance, the energy system dominant in soccer? This is one of the reasons commercials trends have so easily convinced soccer technicians to accept ineffective gadgets, ineffective methods, and the same types of exercises year-round.

In reality, to increase power, speed, and agility, you have to carefully select the types of training, including the loads used.

Research shows that using lighter loads exclusively produces a more modest increase in peak power than is produced by using heavier loads followed by high-velocity training (Aagaard et al, 1994; Verkhoshansky, 1997; Enoka, 2002 and 2015, Duchateau et al, 2021). Indeed, the peak power that a muscle can produce depends directly on gains in maximum strength (Fitts and Widrick, 1996; Seitz, 2014; Schmidtbleicher, 2019; Duchateau et al, 2021).

The same is true for speed. As trainers have known since the 1950s, maximum velocity does not increase unless power is increased first. These findings validate and add more substance to the theory of periodization of strength, allowing us to draw the conclusion that speed, agility, and quickness never increase unless maximum strength is trained first and then converted to power.

Let us explain how the above concepts can be applied in the program of league games (table 6.1).

Strength training during the preparatory phase can be organized as per table 6.1. Please note the months we have referred to correspond to the dates of the Western European leagues. For Brazil, Argentina, and Uruguay, the corresponding months are February and March. Please note that the program starts in the second part of June with the A (adaptation) phase followed by MxS training. The loads should correspond with standard loads for A and MxS.

Table 6.1 Suggested periodization of training and loads of implements

Training details	Preparatory phase		League games
Type of training	A	MxS	Power training Maintain MxS
Load	Medium	Heavy	Medium-light Heavy for MxS
Physiological benefit	Adaptation to medium load	Increase recruitment of FT muscle fibers	Increase discharge rate of FT fibers

During July, most training and loads should be the traditional ones dedicated to power training. In the bottom part of the chart, we have specified the corresponding physiological benefits.

The power exerted during athletic actions depends on the number of active motor units, activated muscle fibers, the FT fibers recruited into the action, and the rate at which they are discharging, producing a high force-to-frequency ratio (Enoka, 2002). The increase in the discharge rate of fast-twitch fibers is achieved by training with lighter loads, either by using less than 50% of 1RM for novice players and between 50% and 60% of 1RM for advanced players (Moritani, 1992; Duchateau and Hainaut, 1998; Morin et al, 2015; Monte et al, 2020) or by using any type of lighter implement (e.g., shots from track and field, power balls, medicine balls) or by performing plyometrics or specific drills for speed, agility, and quickness. Such exercises—performed with maximum power, speed, and quick application of force against the resistance provided by the implement, the pull of gravity, or both—facilitate activation of high-threshold motor units and high frequency of discharge. Such high-velocity exercises are necessary during the second phase when a higher discharge rate of fast-twitch fibers is sought.

Clearly, then, the main scope of strength training for soccer is to continually increase maximum strength so that 50% of 1RM is always higher. This gain, in turn, produces the maximum benefit of increasing peak performance soccer abilities.

Program Design for Power Training

The methodology of training and developing power is relatively rich in opportunities, among them being the isotonic, ballistic, and plyometric methods. The following sections describe these methods and how to implement them in a periodized training plan.

Isotonic Method

The main purpose of power training is to train a player to apply force against resistance, such as the ground, implements, free weights, and medicine balls (MB), as rapidly and forcefully as possible through the entire range of motion. Among the best implements for developing power are free weights, medicine and power balls, and other equipment that can be moved quickly. The weight of the implement used in the isotonic method represents the external resistance a player has to overcome. To defeat the resistance of an implement the player has to apply a superior force. The more the applied force exceeds the external resistance, the faster the acceleration of the implement.

For instance, if a player applies force against an implement equal to 95% of 1RM, they are incapable of generating any acceleration. However, if the same player works on MxS for a year, their strength increases so much that lifting the same weight now equals only 50% of 1RM. Therefore, that same player is now capable of moving the implement dynamically, generating the acceleration necessary to increase power. This difference explains why the periodization of strength requires a maximum strength phase prior to power training. No visible increments of power are possible without clear gains in maximum strength.

MxS is also essential for the early part of a lift or throw. Any implement has a certain inertia, which is its mass or weight. The most difficult part of lifting a heavy implement or throwing an implement explosively is the early part of the motion. To overcome inertia, a player must build a high level of tension in the prime movers. Consequently, the higher a player's MxS, the easier it is to overcome inertia, and the more explosive the start of the movement can be. As the player continues to apply force against the implement, they increase its velocity. As more velocity is developed, less force is necessary to maintain it.

If a player desires to continuously increase an implement's velocity, their limb's speed has to also be increased. However, this is possible only if the player can contract the muscle with high force quickly. As an important physical ability, power is determinant in soccer. Lacking it, a player will never be able to jump higher, run faster, kick the ball more powerfully, or change direction quickly and abruptly.

Do you want to increase players' power? Remember periodization of strength (figure 3.2). Players need not just MxS, but rather to be able to generate MxS at a very high rate, a capacity that can be achieved only through power-training methods.

Training parameters for the isotonic method:

- Load: 60-85% of 1 RM
- Number of exercises: 3-5
- Number of reps per set: 3-5 reps at 50-70 %; 2-4 reps at 70-85%
- Number of sets per exercise: 3-6
- Rest interval: 2-3 minutes
- Speed of execution: Dynamic
- Frequency per week: 2, maximum 3

Soccer players should also attend to safety. When a limb is extended, it should not be snapped. In other words, exercises should be performed dynamically but without jerking the barbell or implement.

Caution: If a player can no longer perform a repetition dynamically, they should stop, even if the set has not been completed. Without dynamic action you are not training power but rather power endurance (discussed at the end of this chapter). Among the essential characteristics of power training are maximum concentration and dynamic action produced by a high recruitment of fast-twitch fiber and its ensuing discharge rate. Both of these physiological benefits are the result of power-training methodology.

Table 6.2 Sample power-training program for players in leagues 1–2

Exercise	Week		
	1	2	3
Calf press	$\dfrac{80 \times 4}{2}$	$\dfrac{85 \times 4}{2}$	$\dfrac{85 \times 4}{2\text{-}3}$
Jump squat	$\dfrac{40 \times 3}{5}$	$\dfrac{45 \times 3}{5}$	$\dfrac{50 \times 3}{5}$
Leg press	$\dfrac{65 \times 4}{3\text{-}5}$	$\dfrac{70 \times 4}{3\text{-}4}$	$\dfrac{80 \times 4}{4\text{-}5}$
Lat pull-down	$\dfrac{50 \times 4}{3}$	$\dfrac{55 \times 4}{3}$	$\dfrac{60 \times 4}{3}$
Weighted crunch	2×12	2×10	2×8

Please adjust the proposed program to the potential of your players.

Ballistic Method

Power training can be applied in different fashions and against a high variety of loads and implements. Therefore, when the resistance of an implement is equal to the force applied by the player, no motion occurs. When, on the other hand, the force applied by the player is higher than the resistance of an implement (e.g., a medicine ball), a dynamic, ballistic motion occurs (kicking or throwing a ball).

During a ballistic action, the player's force has to be applied very quickly. Because of the implement's inertia is high, the beginning of the motion is slower. As the player increases the application of force, the acceleration of the implement also increases throughout the range of motion, culminating in maximum acceleration at the end of motion. Furthermore, the distance the ball is kicked or thrown is proportional to the power applied against it. If you want to generate maximum acceleration, the force applied against the ground has to also be at a maximum, from the beginning to the end of the sprint. This is physics, not personal opinion.

Ballistic power occurs as a result of quick recruitment of fast-twitch muscle fibers, high discharge rate, and effective intermuscular coordination of the agonist and antagonist muscles. For maximum physiological benefits, ballistic exercise should take place after the warm-up, when players are fresh and ready for quality work. If, on the other hand, you intend to improve players' power endurance, plan these activities at the end of the training session, when players are fatigued and performing this type of work is a great challenge.

Training parameters for the ballistic method:

- Load: as per the weight of the implement
- Number of exercises: 2-4
- Number of repetitions per set: 4-6
- Number of sets per training session: 2-5
- Rest interval: 2-3 minutes
- Speed of execution: dynamically
- Training frequency/week: 2-3

For maximum effectiveness of the ballistic training method, the speed of performance is paramount. Every repetition must start dynamically, and the player should try to increase the speed constantly, throughout the motion. This effort enables the involvement of a higher number of fast-twitch motor units. The critical element here is not the number of reps. To increase power, the player need not perform many reps but rather increase the speed of performance, dictated by the quickness of muscle contraction. Therefore, exercises should be performed only as long as quickness is possible. **Repetitions must be discontinued the moment that speed declines.**

The dynamics of power exercises are ensured only as long as a high number of fast-twitch fibers are involved. When the speed of contraction decreases, it signifies a lower participation in the action of the FT fibers. To continue an activity after speed declines is futile since without full activation of fast-twitch motor units, power development is impossible.

The load of ballistic training is dictated by the weight of the implements. Medicine balls weigh from about 1–10 kg, whereas power balls weigh between 1–15 kg.

For maximum effectiveness the number of ballistic exercises must be as low as possible (2–4) in order to facilitate a higher number of sets. A higher number of sets means higher adaptation and a positive transfer of the power needs of soccer players. The selection of exercises has to ensure a specific adaptation, increase physiological benefit, and address to the prime movers used in soccer.

The rest interval between exercises should be as long as necessary to reach full recovery, a guarantee that quality of work is possible in each set. Since ballistic exercises are performed with a partner, a rest interval of 20–30 seconds is already ensured. However, as suggested previously, a longer rest interval is necessary to repeat ballistic actions.

Ballistic training methods can be repeated 2–3 times per week during mid-preparatory phase and twice weekly toward the end of the same training phase and league games. As you decide the frequency of power training, you can also consider other types of speed-power activities, such as maximum accelerations and agility training. Since all these activities tax the same energy system, alactic and lactic, good planning is necessary, not just for training but also for regeneration activities suggested by physiotherapy specialists.

A sample example of a program combining ballistic and maximum acceleration exercises is suggested by table 6.3. This program has been used successfully by some ball players from the United States. Other combinations are also possible, such as technical/tactical and physical, as long as they tax the same energy system. Technical can be combined with other phosphagen types of physical abilities, while tactical can be combined with activities taxing either lactic acid or aerobic.

Table 6.3 A sample program combining ballistic and sprinting

Exercise	Week		
	Week 1	Week 2	Week 3*
Jump squat and medicine ball chest throw	2 × 5	3 × 5	3 × 5
Medicine ball overhead backward throw followed by a 10m backpaddle	2 × 5	3 × 5	3 × 5
Medicine ball chest throw followed by a 20-meter sprint	2 × 5	3 × 5	3 × 5
Medicine ball overhead forward throw	2 × 5	3 × 5	3 × 5
Medicine ball side throw (each side)	1 × 5	3 × 5	3 × 5
Push-up followed by a 15- to 25-meter sprint	3x	4x	5-6x

Data adapted from Bompa, 2006 and 2021.

Plyometric Method

Power training is not a novelty. Simple forms have been used since the ancient Olympic Games. *Jump training*, a term used during the preparation of the U.S. track and field athletes prior to the first modern Olympics, has many similarities with plyometric training.

The term *plyometrics* was first used by Fred Wilt, a U.S. track and field coach, in 1975. Track athletes were also the first to use this method prior to the modern Olympic Games in 1896 in Athens, Greece. At that time, the term used was jump training.

Plyometrics training employs exercises that stimulate the myotatic stretch reflex or the stretch–shortening cycle. These exercises load the muscle in a fast eccentric (lengthening) contraction, followed immediately by a concentric (shortening) contraction. Research in this field has confirmed that if a muscle is quickly stretched before a contraction (pre-stretched), it contracts more forcefully and rapidly (Bosco and Komi, 1980; Schmidtbleicher, 1984 and 2019; Verkhoshansky, 1997; Seiberl et al, 2015; Dorn et al, 2019; Pandy et al, 2021). Therefore, when a player jumps up to head the ball, he lowers the center of gravity first (a stretching action), followed immediately by a powerful contraction when he jumps up.

A plyometric action is performed in three phases (Davis et al, 2015):

1. **Eccentric or pre-stretch**, often called the readiness or pre-loading, is a phase that stretches the muscle-tendon unit in preparation for the next phases.
2. **Amortization**, a rebound phase or an action similar to an elastic recoil, is the time between eccentric pre-stretch and generation of the force to overcome gravity and upward rebound. The shorter the amortization phase, the quicker and more powerful, higher, and longer the take-off of a plyometric action. MxS is one of the most effective methods that can decrease the time of amortization to perform the rebound.
3. **Take-off**, concentric shortening or the actual power-production performance phase, occurs when the elastic properties of pre-stretch muscles are activated to enhance a plyometric performance.

Plyometric methodology and exercises work within complex neural mechanisms. Neural adaptations take place in the body's nervous system to enhance both strength and power (Sale, 1986; Schmidtbleicher, 1992; Enoka, 2015; Pandy et al, 2021). In fact, as already stated, neural adaptations can increase the force of a muscle without increasing its size (Dons et al, 1979; Komi and Bosco, 1978; Sale, 1986; Enoka, 2015; Werkhausen, 2019; Schmidtbleicher, 2019). Therefore, considering these findings, there is no reason for soccer players to be concerned about increasing the size of their muscles.

Please also note that a muscle contracts more forcefully and quickly from a pre- stretched position—and the faster the pre-stretch, the more forceful the concentric contraction. Correct technique is essential. The player must land with the legs slightly bent in order to prevent injury to the knee joints. The shortening contraction should occur immediately after completion of the pre-stretch phase. The transition from the pre-stretch phase should be smooth, continuous, and as swift as possible. Increased contact time indicates fatigue induced by repeated reactive training (Gollhofer et al, 1987; Schmidtbleicher, 2019).

Physiologically, plyometric training is produced in the following sequence:

- quick mobilization of greater innervation activity,
- recruitment of most, if not all, motor units and their corresponding muscle fibers,
- increased firing rate of motor neurons,
- transformation of muscle strength into dynamic, explosive power

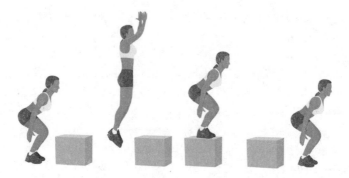

Figure 6.5 An example of power jumps. Variations: directly over; on the box, down, and on again.

Incorporating plyometric training into your training program should be done by considering the following:

- The age and physical development of the player.
- Strength training background. Refrain from exposing young players to plyometrics unless they have previously been exposed to strength training.
- The skills and techniques involved in plyometric exercises.
- Respecting methodical progression (table 6.4) over a long period (2–4 years), progressing from low intensity (levels 5 and 4) to medium intensity (level 3), and then to high intensity (levels 2 and 1).

Plyometric exercises are fun, but also very demanding, as they require maximum concentration and dynamic physical and mental energy. To best assist soccer professionals in organizing plyometric training programs, five intensity zones are proposed (Bompa, 2006). The progression from low to high intensity plyometric exercises should take longer, particularly for young players. You may start such a program from U12 but only with exercises from the bottom of table 6.4.

The two to four years spent incorporating low-impact exercises into the training program of a young player are necessary for the progressive adaptation of the ligaments, tendons, and bones. They also allow for the gradual preparation of the shock-absorbing sections of the player's body, such as the hips and the back muscles: lumbar and intervertebral.

To best serve the needs of power training for soccer, plyometric training has to be game and position specific. Since soccer requires a great degree of horizontal and vertical power, S&C trainers should select specific bounding and hopping drills. This is even more important when you consider the specifics of players' positions in team tactics, such as goalkeepers, defenders, and forwards who often are engaged in a variety of vertical jumps.

Table 6.4 Five intensity levels of plyometric exercise

Classification	Intensity	Exercise	Reps × sets	Reps (or ground contacts) per session	Rest interval (minutes)
1	High intensity	Depth landing: 30–43 in (75–110 cm)	1–5 × 3–6	3–20	5–8
		Depth jump: >28 inches (70 cm)	1–10 × 2–6	3–40	4–8
		Bounding on one leg (or alternating)	40–100 m (or yd) × 2–4	30–150	3–5
2		Drop jump: 16–24 inches (40–60 cm)	3–10 × 2–6	6–40	3–6
		Hurdles: >24 inches (60 cm)	3–12 × 2–6	6–72	3–5
		Bounding on 1–2 legs	5–30 m (or yd) × 2–6	20–60	3–5
		Speed squat (accentuated eccentric); jump squat	3–6 × 2–6	12–24	3–4
3		Hurdles: 16–24 inches (40–60 cm)	6–20 × 2–6	18–80	3–5
4	Low intensity	Box jump: 24–43 inches (60–110 cm)	3–15 × 2–6	12–60	3–5
5		Low hurdles: <12 inches (30 cm)	6–20 × 3–6	18–80	2–3
		Skipping rope	10–30 m (or yd) × 7–15	70–250	1–2
		Medicine ball throws	5–12 × 4–6	20–72	1–3

Data adapted from Bompa, 2006.

Power Training for Soccer

In simple terms, power is defined as the ability to apply force against resistance in the shortest possible time. In soccer, power manifests itself in many ways. Examples include executing a strong push-off against the ground to quickly move in the desired direction, executing a powerful take-off to head the ball towards the goal, and most actions in the penalty area. The player who is the most powerful can also be the most effective during many aspects of the game.

While speed, agility, and quickness depend on the level of power development, power has to be seen as a function of MxS. The higher the force applied against resistance (the ground), the faster a player's action or agility. The source of quickness is force and power. In other words, nobody can be powerful without first being strong.

Improvements in power are achieved during the power-training phase. By using lower loads (50–70% of 1 RM) players are able to perform athletic actions with increased dynamism as a result of increased discharge rate (quickness of muscle contraction) of the fast-twitch muscle.

Another effective means of developing power and quickness of muscle contraction is medicine ball throws and plyometric training, which involves performing a variety of jumps, heaves, hops, and bounding. Power training results in higher overall velocities, increased muscle elasticity, faster reaction times, superior displays of power during specific athletic actions, and improved agility. As noted already, when MxS increases, power increases as well, manifesting itself in displays of high speed, quickness, and agility. Unfortunately, the converse is also true: When MxS decreases, so does power. The decrease of power over the course of a competitive season results in reduced velocity, quickness, and agility. When players begin to show signs of losing speed and agility, strength and power training are effective in getting them back on track.

For the power-training phase, the neuromuscular system is conditioned to increase the discharge rate of FT fibers. In other words, FT fibers are stimulated to contract faster and in larger numbers. A player who has adapted well to power training will be fast, powerful, and able to execute explosive actions with improved agility. The success of power training directly depends on the level of development of MxS, where the FT fibers have been stimulated and conditioned for maximal recruitment into action.

The objective of the power-training phase is to enhance the discharge rate of the FT muscle fibers, which results in a faster, increasingly more agile, and powerful player in all phases of the game. The power-training phase should be planned just prior to the beginning of exhibition or league games to maximize the benefits of this type of training. Table 6.5 gives an example of four-week power training. As you review this suggested program, please keep in mind the following:

- **Jump squat:** Players begin the action in a semi-squat position and holding a medicine ball at chest level. They jump vertically up and should land carefully, in a slight amortization of the eccentric phase. For the purpose of shock absorption during the landing, the first contact should be on the balls of the feet, followed by flexion of the calf, knees, and hips.
- **Medicine ball chest throws followed immediately by a 10 m sprint.** This exercise must be a requirement for goalkeepers, central defenders, and even for strikers. Carefully select the ball weight to reflect the players' abilities and needs.
- **Reactive jumps:** Players jump down from a box 20-75 cm high; they touch the ground first with the balls of the feet before immediately jumping upward, without touching the ground with the heels. The same exercise can be executed with an increased load, such as holding a medicine ball or light dumbbell in each hand.
- **Training sessions per week:** 1-3 depending on age category, background, and facilities, with up to three phases of training: higher fitness sessions during the preparatory phase.
- **Individualized programs:** Adapt the load, number of reps, and sets for each individual player's potential.
- **Proper form for the jump squat:** It is important that athletes perform the jump squat properly to avoid injury. To avoid knee strain, emphasize a cushioned landing (i.e., decelerating upon impact) and always maintaining a vertical upper body.
- **Plyometric exercise level:** Select plyometric exercises according to your players' previous adaptation to similar types of power training.

Table 6.5 Sample three-week training program for dynamic power combined with sprinting speed

Exercise	Week 1	Week 2	Week 3	Rest interval
Jump squat and medicine ball chest throw	2 × 5	3 × 5	3 × 5	3
Forward two-leg jumps over 5 gym benches or low hurdles 1 m apart	2 × 5	3 × 5	3 × 5	2
Medicine ball chest throw followed by 10-meter sprint	2 × 5	3 × 5	3 × 5	3
Medicine ball overhead forward throw	2 × 5	3 × 5	3 × 5	3
Bounding exercise over 10–15 m	2x	3x	3x	2
Two-hand medicine ball throw from chest followed by 20 m sprint	3×	4×	5×	2
Push-up followed by 15-meter bounding jumps	3×	4×	5×	3
Training demand pattern	Low	Medium	High	

Note: Sprinting repetitions may be done in different directions, without or with the ball.

During many power-type activities, such as stop-and-go, changes of direction, or plyometric exercises, muscle fibers contract concentrically (shorten) or eccentrically (lengthen), a physiological manifestation called the stretch-shortening cycle (SSC). Enhanced performance resulting from SSC most likely occurs because of stored elastic energy during the eccentric phase of muscle contraction. Enoka (2015) claims that a strong Achilles tendon can store up to 500 N (50.1 kg), demonstrating the great capability this tendon has to transmit force from the powerful gastrocnemius muscle to the ground to perform a push-off. The same tendon is also responsible for the quick reactivity of a player during landing from a jump and immediately rebounding during a game. Do you want to increase reactivity? Improve MxS and power.

The better the quality of strength training (mostly MxS), the better a player can activate the SSC (Richards et al, 2013; Enoka, 2015; Pandy et al, 2021).

In addition, the above authors suggest that the duration of the SSC and the duration of ground contact can offer information regarding the players' potential:

- Duration of SSC: For fast athletes, it was less than 250 milliseconds; for slow athletes, it was more than 250 milliseconds.
- Duration of foot contact on the ground: For sprinting, contact lasted 80–90 milliseconds; take-off in long jump lasted 140–170 milliseconds; multi-hurdle jumps lasted 150 milliseconds; countermovement jumps lasted 500 milliseconds.

Gastrocnemius anchor

In order to target the prime movers of the leg (mostly the gastrocnemius and soleus muscles), squats, half squats, or step-ups (with a barbell on the shoulders) are often suggested. This approach is wrongly influenced by the sports of weightlifting and powerlifting. During the squat exercise, the most involved joints are the knee extensors (rectus femoris muscles), while the ankles are just partially active. In other words, the most important muscle used during running and agility, the gastrocnemius, is not efficiently targeted in squatting exercises. Effectively targeting the gastrocnemius requires a calf press (at the leg-press machine). Remember that the gastrocnemius contributes more than 50 percent to the force necessary to achieve maximum speed in running, best jumping performance, or maximum quickness in agility actions, while the rectus femoris contributes only 18 percent (Enoka, 2015). Therefore, to efficiently train the muscles needed for maximum speed, running, and agility, use the calf press.

Soccer-Specific Running Power

During the game of soccer players are often in a situation to necessitate an extremely quick start of a sprint, acceleration and deceleration. In fact, deceleration in soccer is as important as acceleration. Both contribute to a player's ability to be agile, to quickly change direction as dictated by the game conditions.

Starting Power

The ability to quickly initiate a sprint, often from standing, or walking, is called starting power. An aggressive sprint directly depends on the player's potential to apply high force against the ground and push the body in the desired direction. The essential physiological capacity to achieve this goal, to quickly start a sprint, is the ability to start the motion very dynamically, explosively, by recruiting in action the highest possible number of fast-twitch fibers. There is a direct relationship between the capacity to recruit high numbers of FT fibers with the level of players' MxS and power. The higher the MxS, the higher the player's potential to recruit FT fibers.

The capacity of a quick start depends on a player's position. If a player is in a pre-stretched position (both knees and hips slightly bent), they can faster activate leg extensors to generate greater power than when relaxed. In this position, the elastic elements of the muscles store kinetic energy that acts like a spring. The power used by first league players should be really high, often 2–2.5 times their own body weight (Bompa and Sarandan, 2023). Higher starting power enables a faster start. Quick action and powerful starts hinge on the elastic, reactive components of the neuromuscular system. The level of MxS achieved during the early part of the preparatory phase can maximize power and agility during the conversion phase, which better improves a muscle's stretch reflex and increases the power of the fast-twitch fibers. Furthermore, the key to starting a motion quickly and powerfully is achievable through isotonic, ballistic power, and plyometric exercises.

Acceleration Power

Acceleration, the ability to quickly increase speed to the highest level possible, directly depends on the player's power, the ability to quickly apply force against the ground. To do so means to have a general, but most importantly, high level of leg power. Without leg power, a player cannot perform the required powerful push against the ground to increase the necessary propulsion power. Obviously, power is an essential attribute to achieving high acceleration.

Recent studies show that ground reaction force during the forward drive is the most important variable in reaching high speed (Weyand et al, 2000; Kyrolainen et al, 2001; Belli et al, 2002; Numella et al, 2007; Brughelli et al, 2011; Morin et al, 2012; Kawamori et al, 2013; Bohm et al, 2015; Schmidtbleicher, 2019; Duchateau et al, 2021). In other words, the players' capacity to accelerate depends on the force of the arms and the legs. Specific strength training for high acceleration will benefit most players, particularly strikers, wings, and full backs.

In any sport requiring fast running, strength is a determinant ability. For instance, if in sprinting in track, the force applied against the ground is three times one's own body weight (Weyand 2010, Seitz et al 2014, Clark and Weyand 2014); similar expectations might be realistic in soccer. For instance, if a player weighs 70 kg, to be very fast he needs to apply a force of 210 kg against the ground. The same weight can easily be applied in calf press. Unfortunately, contemporary training rarely addresses such sporting actions, leading to ineffective exercises used in what should be soccer-specific training.

Deceleration Power

For any player, deceleration is as important as acceleration. This is why soccer players must be able to accelerate and decelerate as quickly as possible in order to accomplish various tactical goals, such as overtaking an opponent or making oneself available to receive a pass. Consequently, soccer players also need the ability to decelerate abruptly, then quickly change their running direction or jump to head the ball. Please remember that the ability to quickly decelerate can create a tactical advantage.

Indeed, deceleration requires strong legs and good biomechanics, such as placing the feet ahead of the center of gravity (the vertical projection of the center of gravity is behind the supporting legs).

The best training methods to improve deceleration are eccentric contraction with high loads, low- to high-impact exercises, and drop or depth jumps from high boxes.

Table 6.6 Sample three-week high-intensity power training for top soccer players

Exercise	Week 1	Week 2	Week 3	Rest interval
MB forward throw between the legs	5x 15	5x 15–20	5x 20–25	3–4
Two-leg jumps over low hurdles	5x over 10 hurdles	6x over 12 hurdles	8x over 15 hurdles	4
Reactive jumps over 50–75 cm boxes	5x	7x	10x	3–4
Bounding 25 meters	4x	5x	5–7x	4
Training demand pattern	Low	Medium	High	

Power Endurance Training

During the soccer game players have to perform repetitive bouts of sprinting at high velocity: high frequency and powerful propulsion. Often, high-velocity sprints are repeated without much rest interval, yet during training some instructors do not demand that players perform 30 strides with maximum force and frequency. (In fact, fake exercises are rarely performed with high speed and power.) This is why sprinting in soccer is ill-prepared to be reproduced with maximum push-off during the game.

When track sprinters cover the classic 100 meters in 10–12 seconds, they have trained to perform powerful leg actions throughout the entire race, not just during the start and the following 6-8 strides, as in fake fitness training in soccer. In a 100-meter race, an athlete takes 48-54 strides, depending on stride length; thus, each leg makes 24-27 contacts with the ground. In each ground contact, the force applied can be more than twice the athlete's body weight. Does anybody analyze sprinting in soccer in the same way?

Power training in soccer is essential if you expect your players to repeat strenuous power activities, after only a few seconds of game interruption. Therefore, to be successful, players need high power output and, equally important, the ability to repeat these actions (power endurance) many times during the game.

Physiologically speaking, there is a difference between a soccer player repeating many short sprints over the duration of a game and a sprinter maintaining high power output for only 30-40 strides. Therefore, a player is repeating an alactic power activity, often without enough recovery time to refill the ATP-CP stores, whereas a sprinter is taxing the anaerobic alactic (phosphagen) energy system during the first part of the race (the first 6-8 seconds). Then, increasingly, the sprinter is taxing the energy system for the rest of a 100 m race. This is why both athletes need power endurance, yet physiologically their types of power endurance differ from each other.

Since power endurance, evidently, is a determinant ability in soccer, we would like to share with your important elements of the methodology for developing power endurance.

Specifically speaking, power endurance in soccer requires a player to apply some 60-70% of maximum strength dynamically throughout the duration of the game. In order to achieve this development of power endurance, a player is required to train 12-30 dynamic reps, with a specific set interval (table 6.5). The needed training can be achieved progressively: start with a low number of reps (10-12) and progress to a higher number of reps (15, 20, 25, or higher). The dual result of applying this methodology should be quite obvious: the ability to cope with fatigue and the capacity to tolerate the build-up of lactic acid induced by performing many reps dynamically.

Training the endurance component of speed has to be not just game specific but also position specific. This goal is accomplished both physiologically, by progressively increasing the number of reps or sets, and psychologically, through a high level of will-power to overcome fatigue and reach optimal mental concentration. This is the reason the number of explosive reps must be high—so that the players learn to tolerate the lactic acid build-up and perform successfully in this condition during the game. Power-endurance methodology will result in maintaining a high rhythm of the game and demonstrate a good physical potential throughout league games. Suggested training parameters for power endurance are summarized in the following list. Power-endurance could be planned parallel with other types of training, preferably after two weeks of power training.

Training parameters suggested for the power endurance method:

- Training phase 3 weeks
- Load 50-70 % of 1RM
- Number of exercises 3-5
- Number of reps per set 12-30
- Number of sets per exercise 3-5
- Rest interval 3-4 minutes
- Speed of execution Dynamic
- Frequency per week 2

Training Goalkeepers

As the last defender of their team, goalkeepers are always a special concern for the coach. This is why many teams have a special coach just for training the goalies. However, are goalkeepers properly trained? Are coaches training the specific abilities needed to be a successful goalkeeper?

Have you ever seen how keepers are trained? In most cases, training a goalkeeper means hitting the ground many, many times during a training session! Is this what actually makes a goalie well-trained and successful?

Let's analyze the physical attributes needed for a goalkeeper.

Power. A well-trained goalkeeper has to dive, jump, and move quickly in many directions to block or punch a ball, all of which require power. Yes, **leg power**. Any action performed by a goalkeeper starts with applying leg force against the ground to move the player in the desired direction. Therefore, when you plan a training program for a goalkeeper you have to start from the legs up. Not to mention the essential ability to react quickly to prevent a goal. As already mentioned above, all these physical abilities have an important source: MxS. Yes, MxS!

Core strength, abdominals, low back, and intervertebral muscles. During the game a goalkeeper is often on the ground, and must raise the trunk, and the body in general, to stand up and move where they need to. To be ready to perform all these actions, goalies also need a well-trained midsection. Hopefully, we have already demonstrated the importance of MxS for everything that requires speed, power, and agility. This is also the case with goalies.

Reaction time, choice reaction, and movement time to assist the player in performing all the above-mentioned actions (chapter 7). To best and effectively train a goalie and to achieve the above physical objectives you have to create a periodization plan (figure 6.2). The proposed periodization plan is very similar to the one you have to design for the entire team. Training MxS, followed by power training, will make the goalie push against the ground with a higher number of fast-twitch muscle fibers and, as a result, move faster or jump higher to catch or punch a ball. Therefore, good MxS training secures the physiological base to equip the goalie with the essential physical attributes to fulfill their role on a soccer team.

Preparatory		League games
A	MxS, P, Ag, R	Maintain MxS, P, Ag, R

A = adaptation; P = power; Ag = agility; R = reactivity

Figure 6.2 Periodization of training for a goalkeeper.

Note: The training methods proposed for the development of MxS and power for all players have to be used for the goalkeeper as well. However, more attention should be dedicated to the development of reactivity, an essential ability needed for these players. Goalkeepers' training can be enriched by using reactive ball exercises for the development of reactivity and reaction time.

Conclusions

Power training is a determinant ability for any player who wants to apply force against the ground to perform fast, agile, and quick feet. However, the level of power directly depends on MxS, or the ability of a player to recruit as many muscle fibers as possible. However, a high level of power is an impossible task without the ability of those same muscle fibers to increase the discharge rate.

Please remember that powerful, fast actions are performed by muscles. Consequently, if you want to make a player fast and agile, you have to train the specific muscles (prime movers) to be capable of executing the required actions and moves.

There is no other method apart from periodization of strength that can improve power, speed, and agility.

CHAPTER 7
CONVERTING MXS INTO
SOCCER-SPECIFIC SPRINTING SPEED

KEY POINTS

- What Makes a Soccer Player Fast? Guidelines for Speed Training
- Principles of Speed Training: A Condensed Form Program Design for Sprinting Speed
- Factors Affecting Sprinting Speed Exercise Selection: What Works and What Doesn't

In the game of soccer, speed, or sprinting speed, is a multidirectional athletic activity, since running is performed in all directions during the course of a game. In addition to running forward, soccer players must often move sideways and backward (backpedaling) or are required to pivot, zigzag, stop and go, cut, turn, and change direction in response to the dynamics of the game.

The world of athletics offers many examples regarding the maximum speed some athletes can generate during games or competitions. Let us share with you some incredible results (based on the information provided by Mero, 1992; Weyand et al, 2000; Weyand et al, 2010; Horsfield, 2015; Trackspikes Co, UK, 2018):

- Usain Bolt, sprinter: 44.7 km/hour
- Leo Messi, soccer: 32.5 km/h
- Cristiano Ronaldo, soccer: 33.6 km/h
- Tyreek Hill, American football (Kansas Chiefs): 36.6 km/h
- Ball velocity in soccer: Men: 26.4. m/s, women: 22.0 m/s

What Makes a Soccer Player Fast?

Good question! In a simple world, there are two answers only:

1. genetics
2. MxS

In the first case, genetics refers to the proportion between the fast-twitch (FT) and slow-twitch (ST) muscle fibers. If a player was lucky to inherit a parent's higher number of FT, this person can be your fast player. Otherwise, there are many other sports which do not require a great amount of speed. Since you cannot alter your genetic code, the only option to become faster is to increase your MxS.

Have you ever asked yourself why some cars are faster than others? To best understand the role of maximum strength (MxS) in soccer, consider the following analogy. Compare two cars: one is an ordinary car, the other a sports car. Why is the sports car faster? Because of its shape? Or because the sport car has a stronger engine, and a higher level of horsepower (HP)? Remember: the stronger the engine, the faster the car.

If a car with a powerful engine can generate high velocity, why don't we accept that a soccer player with powerful engine—a high level of MxS—can be fast simply because they are very strong and can apply high force against the ground to push the body forward faster?

Strength training in soccer is still a confusing issue and, in some cases, in the infancy stage. Amazingly, there are still some soccer professionals who believe that strength is not needed in soccer. Again, if the engine is the reason a car is faster than the other, we have to also accept that MxS is the engine that makes a player faster than others.

Remember, the stronger the player's engine (MxS), the faster and more agile the player.

Fast athletes are also very strong. Ben Johnson, the Olympic Champion in 100m at the Seoul Olympics, was able to do a leg press with 300kg whereas for a calf press he was able to press 320 kg. Ben could press heavier loads, but a patella irritation made him stop at 270 kg (from Charly Francis, Ben's coach, and Tudor O. Bumpa's personal diaries).

A high level of speed is achieved only when a player is capable of *applying high force against the ground in the shortest period of time*, particularly during the propulsion phase (i.e., the push-off against the ground). If you want to jump high to head a ball, you have to apply high force against the ground to overcome the force of gravity.

The same is true for speed: ***the ability to generate high velocity is proportional to the force applied against the ground***. This is the only way to generate high **sprinting** speed in soccer. You have to ***apply the highest* force in the minimum time,** meaning the **shortest duration of the foot contact on the ground**, or around 100 milliseconds (mls).

Duration of ground contact (Weyand et al 2010):

- Top sprinters: 90–120 mls
- Good sprinters/runners: < 150 mls
- Mediocre sprinters: > 200–250 mls

Duration of ground contact is an essential element in sprinting and jumping sporting actions. One can apply quick force in the shortest period of time only if the player's MxS is high:

- It is quite impossible to have a fast player without short duration of foot contact on the ground. The longer the duration of foot contact on the ground, the slower the player. Imagine two players, side by side. One can apply force against the ground very fast, and the duration of foot contact is 150 mls. The other player needs 170 mls to leave the ground. Who is the faster player? The player whose duration of the foot on the ground is shorter, 150 mls. In a sprint of 20 meters, covered in 12 strides, the faster player has a gain of 240 mls. Fast foot action, fast application of force against the ground, is made by the calf muscles, particularly the gastrocnemius muscle.
- It is impossible to have a short duration of foot contact on the ground without MxS. The rapid application of force against the ground is proof that only the players with strong gastrocnemius/soleus muscles can have a fast propulsion phase and a short duration of foot contact on the ground and be a fast player.

(For more information on the topic please refer to the works of Ekblom, 1986; Sale, 1986; Schmidtbleicher, 1984 and 2019; Neptune and Sasaki, 2005; Bloomfield et al, 2007; Hamner et al, 2010; Weyand et al, 2010; Dorn et al, 2012; Clark and Weyand, 2014; Seitz et al, 2014; Bohm et al, 2015; Colyer et al, 2018; Werkhausen et al, 2019; Dolci et al, 2020; Ferris and Hawkins, 2020; Duchateau et al, 2021; Pandy et al, 2021.)

Principles of Running Technique: A Condensed Form

For purposes of practicality, speed training for soccer has two phases: acceleration and maximum speed. During acceleration (10-15 meters), players have to progressively and very quickly reach maximum speed. After that, players have to maintain maximum speed for the duration of the action.

To achieve maximum speed the ankles, hips, and knees must be fully extended. This triple joint extension demonstrates not only good leg, hip, and core power but also optimal technique. A strong body leads to good form, and good form leads to faster performances.

Although sprinting in soccer is often different than in track and field, the general mechanics of running are similar. The only time a soccer player has similar track technique is during longer, forward sprints, such as those performed by wingers or side midfielders. Soccer players are not always the most effective runners because team sport training seldom works on the correct mechanics of running. As a result, some players use a very inefficient running technique.

Do you want to produce fast players? Apply MxS methodology using exercises such as leg press and calf press on leg-press machines. These exercises effectively target the gastrocnemius muscle, are the powerhouse exercise for sprinting, and are incomparably safer than weight-lifting exercises!

The proper running technique contains the following four phases:

1. **The propulsion phase.** To drive the body forward as fast as possible, the player applies force by pushing the foot and leg against the ground powerfully and quickly (figure 7.1). To improve sprinting speed, a player has to first increase leg force using the triple extensors muscles (calf, knees, and hips), that directly assist also in also increasing the legs' propulsion. As compared to other muscles, gastrocnemius and soleus are the main contributors to an athlete's speed (51%), followed by hamstrings, quadriceps, and gluteus maximus (18%) (Enoka, 2015). All these muscles together apply a force 3-5 times the athlete's body weight (Sasaki and Neptune, 2006; Hemner et al, 2010; Wayand, 2010; Clark and Wayand, 2014; Schmdtbleicher 2019).

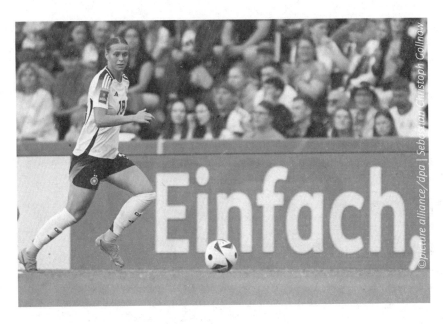

Figure 7.1 The propulsion (push-off) phase of the running step. Observe the angle of the push-off ankle (left leg) as demonstrating good push-off efficiency.

2. During **the drive phase**, the lead leg propels forward, so that the thigh is almost parallel to the ground. The forward-swinging arm is also moving along the body, with the hand reaching shoulder height. The fast movement of the legs is always determined by the arm drive, unlike some artificial drills, such as fast running on the spot. Remember: stronger leg power and quicker application of force against the ground means faster sprinting speed.

3. **The foot landing phase**: As soon as the foot strikes the ground, it begins to quickly move underneath the body, followed by the recovery phase. To ensure that the calf muscles do not collapse at the instant of landing, the ankle has to be locked and stiff. This is achieved only by increasing foot and ankle strength. The higher the force, the higher the reactivity of foot and ankle muscles. An effective criterion to evaluate ankle's force is to observe the landing technique. If the heel of the foot touches the ground, it means the calf muscles are not strong enough to maintain ankle stiffness during landing, and, as a result, it prolongs the duration of the contact phase. A longer duration of contact phase means a decrease in the speed of a

player. Calf stiffness is proportional to the MxS of gastrocnemius, soleus, and tibialis anterior. Please also remember that landing amortization is performed eccentrically by the calf muscles, whereas the reactive action (push-off, jumps) is done by the same muscles but concentrically.

4. **The recovery phase**: To shorten the recovery phase, the opposing arm is quickly driven forward. Therefore, maximum speed is achieved not only by the force of the propulsion muscles but also by the quickness of contraction of the knee flexors of the hamstring muscles. Hamstrings are important for the forward ground reaction (Morin et al, 2015). Hamstrings also have a higher innervation per square centimeter than the quadriceps muscles (Enoka, 2015), resulting in high reactivity and speed of contraction, and, as such, higher incidents of injuries (at the upper junction of hamstrings). The likelihood of injury can be decreased by improving their strength! Among the best exercises are Nordic curls and reverse leg presses.

When analyzing running technique, look for the following elements:

- To reach high velocity, players should have a shorter duration of contact phase with the ground. Therefore, they must run on the balls and toes of the feet.
- The contact phase of the supporting leg remains as short as possible. A prolongation of the contact phase demonstrates a lack of power and reactivity.
- The fastest players generally have a contact phase between 180 and 210 milliseconds (mls). Elite sprinters come closer to 90–120 mls (Bompa and Francis, 1995; Weyand et al, 2000).
- The torso remains as erect as possible. The hand of the driving arm comes up, close to face level.
- Shoulder and facial muscles are relaxed. Any tension of these muscles reflects unnecessary contraction, rigidity, and unnecessary energy expenditure.
- The hips are high, legs fully extended, as a demonstration of an effective propulsion (push-off) phase. If this position is incorrect, it means the push-off leg did not complete its forceful action, and it may be impossible to reach maximum speed.
- The height of the center of gravity (CG) changes constantly for soccer players depending on their pattern of movement. When a player decelerates and then accelerates in another direction, the CG lowers progressively during

deceleration (the lowest point occurring when the player actually stops), while the CG rises progressively during acceleration (the highest point occurring during maximum acceleration). The CG will also adjust sideways, forward, and backward depending on the player's running pattern. Since team sports tend to be very dynamic and interactive, players will rarely run with a pure sprinting style, except in situations where they run in a relatively straight line or along a slightly curvilinear path.

- A player achieves maximum speed only after accelerating for at least 10-15 m. To reach maximum velocity, players must react quickly and apply maximum force against the ground to achieve a strong push-off. Stronger players achieve their maximum speed faster than their weaker counterparts.
- To improve running efficiency, athletes should constantly be aware of a correct, good running form.
- A strong arm drive is crucial for achieving optimal running technique. Arms are driven backward and forward up to face level. The leg-driving frequency increases as the rate of the arm drive increases.
- The thigh of the driving leg (the left leg in figure 10.4) should swing up to the horizontal; from this point, the foot of the same leg is projected forward and downward, towards the ground.
- The position of the body remains vertical, and the eyes focus ahead as the ball of the foot contacts the ground with a brushing action. The foot strikes the ground quickly, coming underneath the body as the body moves forward.
- As the body moves forward, the other leg (right) is driven forward. The left leg now pushes against the ground, projecting the body forward.
- These actions are repeated as long as the sprint lasts in an unbroken rhythmical cycle. During this cycle, both legs have alternate supporting and driving functions, while the rhythmical movements of the bent arms assist the stride rhythm.

Note: These technical requirements are more specific to track athletes than soccer players. However, to apply the above technical cues to soccer is difficult for two reasons:

1. Except for wingers and side midfielders, other players rarely have the opportunity to perform long sprints (35-40 m).
2. During the game, changes of direction occur so often that players do not have the time and space to apply these cues.

Factors Affecting Sprinting Speed

Many factors influence speed development, including genetics, movement speed, power, technique, concentration and will-power, muscle elasticity, and joint flexibility.

Unlike other motor abilities such as strength and endurance, where athletes are able to achieve significant improvements after sufficient training without possessing outstanding talent, speed is determined largely by a player's own genetic code and requires a greater degree of natural talent.

Inherited factors such as the mobility of nervous processes, the quick alternation between excitation and inhibition, and the capacity to regulate neuromuscular coordination affect motor frequency and efficiency, which are both determinant factors in developing speed. For best success in sprinting speed, consider the following factors that might have a negative effect on your quest to develop fast players:

• **Strength and power.** The force of a muscular contraction (i.e., the capacity of a player to display force) is a major determining factor for performing fast movements in most sports. During training and games, external resistance to player movements comes from a variety of sources, including gravity, the environment (water, wet field, snow, wind), and opponents. Players require power to overcome these opposing forces through enhanced muscular capabilities. Players must often perform a skill quickly and repeat it with the same quality many times during a game. As a result, players must complement the development of power with the development of power endurance during speed training, which will allow players to perform many fast and quick actions for the duration of a game.

Note: When a genetically talented player for speed is also exposed to a highly methodical strength-training program, you may have a high-class player on your hands!

- **Psychomotor abilities.** Reaction time, dexterity, and visual skills are examples of largely inherited abilities that are important for successful performance in soccer. These skills are outwardly manifested in ball control, precise receiving and passing, and accuracy in shooting. Furthermore, among the numerous psychomotor abilities, the capacity to react quickly is considered one of the most cherished abilities in soccer. It represents the time needed to initiate a response to a given stimulus during game situations. Gaining control of the ball from the opponent or goalies responding to the actions of offensive players are examples of the incredible importance of reaction time.

- **Movement time.** This is generally considered to be the elapsed time between the first overt movement of a response and the completion of that action. Achieving fast movement time depends on the ability of muscles to contract quickly and powerfully, which is essential in soccer. The faster a limb is able to move, the faster a player can get into position to shoot, block, retrieve, or intercept the ball.

- **Technique and concentration.** When proper technique is used to perform skills, speed performance is improved by shortening the time of limb actions, correctly positioning the center of gravity, and using energy more efficiently. Proper form, particularly in sprints over 20 m, enables players to carry out skills effortlessly and with a high degree of accuracy, coordination via the relaxation of antagonistic muscles.

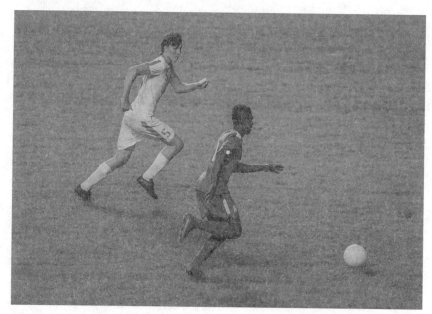

Figure 7.2 High sprinting speed in soccer can have a determinant role in many aspects of the game, particularly as a tactical weapon, with its maximum effectiveness being during counterattacks and transition from defense to offense and offense to defense.

Figure 7.2 exemplifies a good technique during sprinting and ball control (player in the white jersey). Note the position of the knee drive, intended to go high up diagonally, increasing stride length. However, stride length can be influenced by many factors of the game, including the defender's distance. The arms' drive is used to increase arm frequency and improve sprinting speed.

Note: This technique is achievable only in direct, maximum sprinting conditions during the game. In all other sprinting conditions, the body and arms might be at different angles. Straight-line sprinting is the fastest but not often possible during the game. On the other hand, bend running, often performed by wingers, is 2–3% slower than straight sprinting (Churchill et al, 2015). As with other aspects of sprinting speed, the effectiveness of bend running can be increased via improving the legs' force and agility.

Strong concentration enables players to mobilize their nervous processes more effectively and maintain maximum alertness. Therefore, before any speed drill or exercise, players must be prepared to participate with maximum concentration as well as the will to go faster.

Guidelines for Sprinting Speed Training

As you are planning your sprinting speed training methodology for your team, please consider the following five important variables: intensity, duration, volume, frequency, and rest intervals.

Intensity

Intensity represents the qualitative elements of soccer training such as sprinting speed, agility, reactivity, and also speed endurance. Improvements in sprinting speed are highly effective when running technique is good, relaxed, its physiological foundation is based on MxS and power, and when running intensity is in the area of 90-100% of maximum. The highest sprinting gains are usually made when players are rested, when fatigue from other activities does not hinder the development of maximum sprinting speed or quickness. Therefore, this usually occurs immediately after the warm-up following one or more days of rest, or low-intensity training. Since training for maximum speed is very demanding mentally and physically, adequate rest between training days and repetitions is essential.

The appropriate intensity levels are determined by several factors:

Drill intensity. For maximum training benefits, technical fitness drills used in soccer must be performed with high power and with a very dynamic rhythm. To avoid undesirable fatigue, S&C trainers have to properly monitor the drills' intensity, number of repetitions, their duration, and the rest intervals between them. To effectively facilitate regeneration, technical coaches should carefully alternate energy systems, both during the training session and the week (microcycle).

Rhythm of games and drills. Games and drills can be very taxing, both physically and psychologically. While these factors can be controlled during training, the pace of a game depends on the tactics used by both teams. If your players are not ready to play against other teams that use a fast game pace, your team is unlikely to be successful.

Number of games per week and their schedule cannot be controlled. However, to ready your team for varied, unpredictable game conditions, read about the model training methodology presented in chapter 10. It is generally not a good idea to plan exhibition games during the season, unless you have only one game scheduled in a week. Therefore, exhibition games should be planned mostly during the second half of the preparatory phase, pre-league games, or during the eventual interruption of your league games.

Minutes played by the best players have to be closely monitored by the technical coach, regarding training demand, and to avoid injuries. During the course of a game, most coaches heavily rely on the most talented players on a team. This is why technical coaches have to create individualized training programs, and, if necessary, reduce their training intensity following some games. During the first post-game training sessions, fatigued players should not be exposed to highly demanding training sessions, but rather to a regeneration/recovery period for the body and mind. Negligence in this respect may result in undesirable high-level fatigue or exhaustion.

Players' rates of recovery are rarely the same. Consequently, the level of aerobic endurance and the position on the team have to be considered when the coach plans the recovery-regeneration strategy and physiotherapy techniques. Coaches and medical staff should always consider all these factors, including players' levels of fatigue and rates of recovery, when they apply their recovery strategy. Similarly, the morning immediately after game day may be used for recovery, regeneration, and physiotherapy techniques. Even the post-game evening may be planned according to players' physical and psychological status, and, therefore, be a less demanding training session.

Social and psychological stressors have to constantly be monitored and controlled, including their sources, such as players' intimate relationships, lifestyles, peer pressure, or even professional engagements. An analysis of these factors should also be considered when planning a training session, leading to careful manipulation of the volume and intensity of training sessions. A stressed player may have some difficulties tolerating a high-volume training session. At the same time, stress may affect players' concentration levels, and, in this case, the coach should not plan a high-intensity session. Therefore, coaches must identify these external stressors and discuss them privately with each player. Stress-free players are the most effective players.

Sprinting Distance and Duration

Training distance and the duration of a repetition has to consider the distance needed by a player to accelerate and maintain maximum sprinting speed. In other words, you need to plan a maximum distance of at least 20 m. If the distance is less than 20 m, your players work only on the acceleration, not on developing maximum speed. On the other hand, if the duration of a drill is too short (4-8 seconds), as is the case in most contemporary training, the player does not reach maximum quickness, instead only improving short duration quickness, taxing just the phosphagen (alactic) energy system. Therefore, side midfielders and wingers should train longer distances, such as 30–40 m, and participate in drills lasting 15-20 seconds or longer. In the latter case, players are taxing the glycolytic, lactic acid energy system, rarely trained in contemporary training methods.

Training Volume: Training volume is the quantitative element of training: the duration, distance, or amount of work performed during training or games. Since speed training places a great strain on the central nervous system (CNS) and the neuromuscular system, training volume for sprinting speed should remain low (20–30 minutes), depending on the duration, number of repetitions of the selected drills, distance, and number of repetitions.

Training Frequency: As compared to endurance training, the energy spent during speed training is relatively low, but energy expenditure per time unit is very high, demonstrating, therefore, why fatigue sets in so quickly during speed-training sessions. Therefore, players should repeat maximum intensities no more than 6-8 times per session or 2-3 times per week depending on the game schedule.

Number of Repetitions: Specific training to improve maximum sprinting speed is age related and best achieved by performing 6-8 repetitions of 20-40 m, with a rest interval of 3-4 minutes. If the coach plans a higher number of repetitions (8-12 or more), players will also improve speed-endurance levels, and the capacity to tolerate the build-up of lactic acid. This form of training is important particularly for wingers, midfielders, and forwards, all of whom periodically require quick and repeated accelerations throughout the game.

Rest Interval: Since high-intensity training, sprinting speed, and agility is very taxing, players require a longer rest interval (RI) to ensure the replenishment of the high amount of energy fuels used: 2 to 3 minutes RI for the phosphagen energy and 3 to 4 minutes for drills taxing the glycolytic energy system. If the RI results only in partial recovery, the players do not have the time to completely remove lactates from the system and, therefore, may have some difficulty to complete the training plan. Occasionally, however, coaches should specifically plan training sessions where players have to increase the capacity to tolerate high lactic acid build-up, and, as a result, be ready for very difficult games.

Program Design for Developing Sprinting Speed

The method for training sprinting speed is a relatively simple running technique but physiologically is very demanding, with high-energy expenditures per time unit. Success in sprinting speed highly depends on players' MxS and power. Consequently, to train specific sprinting speed in soccer you must use technical, tactical drills, maximum velocity sprinting drills as well as well-designed and periodized MxS and power training. Training both sprinting speed and power is essential for improving your players' sprinting.

Repetition Method: The Essential Training Formula for Sprinting Speed

Repetition training is a traditional training method that has been used in track and field since the late 1800s and can be implemented in soccer training to great effect. For best improvements in sprinting speed over a given distance, or the quickness in technical and tactical drills, an activity must be repeated several times at a high velocity, over 90% of maximum speed.

For highest training success, during repetition training, players must use maximum concentration and must be focused on performing each repetition at the described speed. Maximum concentration will help players reach superior speed, good technique, and neuromuscular coordination.

Note: Rigidity in running is normally expressed by facial grimaces, making it easy to tell who runs in a relaxed manner and who does not.

Specific Training Methods

Technical and tactical drills are an important part of soccer-specific training. These drills have to be game- and position-specific exercises, done with and without the ball, keeping in mind tactical implications and the principles of energy systems.

The ability to run quickly, to abruptly accelerate in various parts of the game is not sufficient. For most players, acceleration–deceleration coupling, or the ability to slow down quickly after running with maximum velocity, is as important in soccer as the ability to accelerate quickly. Since players rarely accelerate in a straight line, they must become accustomed to executing many game-specific actions and tactical maneuvers during training, including turns, pedaling backward and to the side, direction changes, and stop-and-go movements.

The distance covered during sprinting speed and technical and tactical drills (table 7.1) should be 10–30 m and longer, up to 50 m, for wingers and midfielders, repeated several times, depending on age category. Regardless of how far a player runs at maximum speed, special sessions of speed training should be organized that incorporate elements of maximum acceleration and deceleration and are combined with agility drills. These types of training programs improve acceleration and deceleration but also elements of athleticism (please refer to the agility section).

Table 7.1 Selected methods for speed training, distance of activity, number of repetitions, and duration of rest interval

Training form	Activity distance (m/yd)	Number of repetitions	Rest interval (min)	Speed training sessions per week
Nonspecific drills				
Maximum accelerations	10-30	6-10	3-4	1-2
Maximum speed	20-50	4-8	3-4	1-2
Soccer-specific drills				
Acceleration	10-30	4-6	2	2-3
Deceleration	10-20	4-6	2	2
Stop and go	10-20	4-6	2	2
Acceleration, direction changes, etc.	10-30	4-8	2	2-3

Training suggestions in table 7.1 may also be modified as follows:

- One or two days per week, train maximum acceleration sprints, maximum speed training, and acceleration with changes of direction.
- Two days per week, train acceleration–deceleration and stop-and-go sprints.
- Since speed training can be extremely taxing, both mentally and physically, it is important to monitor the amount and type of training used during each training session. A general guideline would be to incorporate two to four types of training per session, two or three times per week, depending on the player's skill level, physical potential, and game schedule. The balance of training should focus on technical and tactical work.
- Also, make note of the suggested number of speed sessions per week. Several of the suggested forms of training can be planned for the same day, setting aside only two or three days of highly taxing maximum speed training per week. By using the concept of alternating energy systems in training, your players will be able to cope more effectively with the fatigue induced by high-intensity training.

Nonspecific Training Methods

Most nonspecific speed-training methods were originally borrowed from track and field but adjusted to the needs of soccer. For the purposes of simplicity and improved efficiency, we are proposing seven types of training, all specific to soccer.

Maximum acceleration, or the capacity to quickly run in the desired direction, is not just a game necessity, but can often have a tactical benefit by allowing a player to quickly explode away from an opponent towards a specific place to receive the ball. To maximize speed, players should emphasize a powerful arm drive in the direction of the run. As the arm drives forward quickly, it stimulates a subsequent knee drive of the opposite leg in the same direction. In other words, sprinting speed is initiated by the arms and the high rate of leg frequency. Move the arms first, and the legs will follow!

The repetition method for improving maximum acceleration has to be performed from different positions: standing, walking, backpedaling, and so on. For variation, you can use maximum acceleration drills by combining them with running in various directions (e.g., zigzag, slalom, sideways), or even combining them with a specific action. The only limit is your imagination! Acceleration drills can be repeated for 10–40 m, 6–8 times or higher as per the player's physical potential. Suggested rest interval: 2–3 minutes.

Maximum sprinting speed is always achieved after a short period of acceleration. The more vigorous your acceleration, the more effective your maximum sprinting speed. The purpose of maximum sprinting speed training is to constantly make your players faster than the opponents. Information regarding speed training is presented in table 7.1. For training maximum speed, you can also use the following training methods.

Note: Remember, maximum speed always depends on reaction time and MxS.

Anticipation drills help players to be one step ahead of the opponent, often giving them the ability to read the game, react to the situation, and take best tactical position. and Previous experience may allow players to quickly identify familiar game cues and respond quickly and effectively. It is also important to expose players to model-training methodology (chapter 10), and apply drills that can replicate specific game conditions and ready the team for the next game.

Decision-making drills exercise the critical ability to make quick decisions. A fast game always shortens the time available to make quick decisions. Many players are exposed to a high variety of stimuli, from player movement and its direction, to speed and direction of the ball. With all these stimuli to contend with, players must be alert and attentive at all times to be able to read the game effectively and to respond accordingly in a short period of time. Players' experience can have an important impact on the quickness of decision-making process. To enhance all the above processes, you are advised to employ the methodology of model training (chapter 10) during training and games.

Note: Obviously, not all forms of training have to be used in the same training session. Because of its demanding characteristics, maximum speed is usually trained separately from other types of training, along with tactical training taxing the aerobic energy system. However, always beware of the rest interval you prescribe for your players.

Speed training can be trained in a high variety of diagrams and from all possible positions a player experiences during the game. Figure 7.3 depicts some of the common symbols used to represent various movements incorporated into speed and quickness drills. A multitude of possibilities exist for developing speed and quickness drills, especially since they can be performed with or without a ball or puck and can be designed to be sport and position specific.

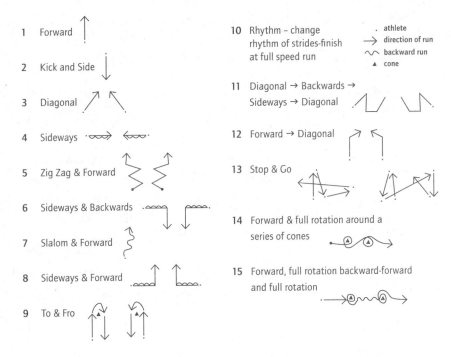

Figure 7.3 Selected running or skating patterns for the development of specific speed. Running or skating may be initiated from standing, kneeling, lying down, or any other position a player may experience during a game. Use markers on the floor, field, or arena to suggest your selected pattern.

Exercise Selection for Sprinting Speed Training: What Works and What Doesn't

All soccer players have the same desire: to be fast and play the game with a high rhythm. This is a highly respected desire, except that some elements of contemporary training cannot deliver this intent, since some players are being poorly trained, at times with inappropriate methods. Strength training is a travesty! Unless players increase MxS, sprinting speed will not be increased. Remember that the acceleration of a body is directly proportionate to the force applied against the ground. No additional force, no additional sprinting speed.

The same applies when it comes to increasing the rhythm of the game: agility drills of 4–8 seconds will never result in increased rhythm of the game. Instead, try specific endurance training (chapter 9).

Speed, agility, and quickness training (SAQ). The promoters of SAQ training claim that by jogging over rings, or around different markers and accessories, such as cones, speed ladder, and so on, players can improve SAQ. This type of training has taken fitness training in soccer in a wrong direction. Please consider the following comments and make your own decision:

- All SAQ drills are very short, 4–8 seconds, taxing the alactic/phosphagen energy system. Please also remember that the alactic energy system supplies only 15% of the energy needed during a game.
- Why is so much time and energy spent on only 15% of the energy required during a game? When do you train the other 85%? Some elements of contemporary training have a minimal physiological benefit. Just an impersonation of what top players should do.
- The kind of speed done during SAQ drills is jogging, not maximum speed. One needs a great deal of imagination to claim that these drills improve speed. Only high-intensity drills and strength training can increase sprinting speed.
- Deceleration in soccer is as important as acceleration. When you can stop faster than your direct opponent, you have a tactical advantage. Both are elements of agility, yet you will rarely see drills specifically planned to improve deceleration.
- Often, the SAQ drills are just mimicking high speed and agility. You should create drills where the speed has to be 90–100 % of players' potential. When players adapt to this type of speed, they will also be able to duplicate it during the game.
- During some drills, players pretend to also work on leg and hip flexibility. As visible in the SAQ drills, the feet are lifted only to the knee level! Please do not call it flexibility training! Do not waste players' time and energy with useless activities.
- Please research the training programs done by top soccer teams:
  » They rarely have a system of training based on the principles of the physiology of soccer.
  » For best physiological adaptation and benefit, alternate energy-system training to facilitate players' recovery and regeneration (see chapter 10).
  » There is no training system based on periodization, from strength to speed and agility.

» Some instructors do not plan the time and exercises to prevent injuries by strengthening muscles, ligaments, and tendons.

- If you do not train the lactic acid and aerobic energy systems, on what basis do you expect your players to play with a high rhythm during the game?

- In spite of some of their conceptual misunderstanding, some types of SAQ training have some merit, such as training variety.

Selected Suggestions for SAQ Training:

- Use the principles of energy systems to train and improve all the physiological aspects of the game (maximum speed, agility, and specific endurance).

- Do not use the terms speed or explosiveness for something performed with 30–40% of player potential. This is misleading, to say the least.

- This type of training has modest physiological benefits.

- The duration of SAQ drills has to be properly planned and the rest interval between them has to be calculated as per the principles of energy-system training.

- Use drills for all three energy systems to ensure complete physiological adaptation as per the requirements of the physiology of soccer.

For a comparison between contemporary mentality and that of the great Javier Zanetti (age 50), who played 858 games in top leagues (Inter Milano 1995–2014, 145 games for Argentina), winning 16 titles, including one World Cup for Clubs, we would like to quote one of his adages: "Every Monday I did strength training. This was one of my secrets of longevity and of being an injury-free player. Speed is not gained by sprinting but rather by the force you acquire in the gym."

Low hurdles (figure 7.4) are purported to train hips' flexibility and speed. When low hurdles are used, the players are running for a few meters and clear, jumping over low- to middle-height hurdles. But considering the height of the feet and the angle between the trunk and legs, it's hard to believe that this exercise might result in any real development of hip flexibility or sprinting speed. The hurdle walkover is promoted as a method for training leg strength and flexibility. In reality it develops neither since simple walking over a hurdle can be done by any U12 player. If a U12 player can do this exercise, it means it does not challenge a more advanced player, and if there is no physiological challenge, there is no training benefit. Another ineffective exercise promoted by popular gym-training trends.

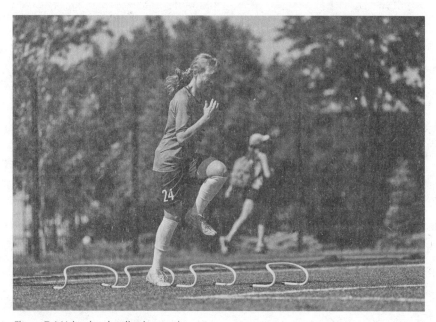

Figure 7.4 Using low hurdles in practice.

Occasionally, in soccer, a player needs to lift the foot up to shoulders/head height with ease to control a high ball (figure 7.5). Naturally, players must train hip and leg flexibility to do this without risk of injury. However, flexibility training in soccer rarely achieves its goal.

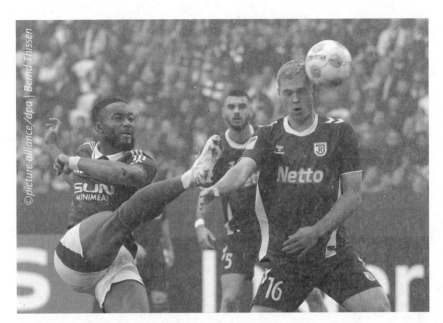

Figure 7.5 An example of what good hip flexibility actually means.

Speed ladders (figure 7.6) have become very popular among fitness trainers, where the scope of training is the development of agility, reactivity, and rapid foot movements. There is a high array of exercises one can do on a speed ladder. However, there are three major problems with these exercises:

1. They are used for ages 6–36.
2. The same moves are repeated over and over with the same ladder and the same force application against the ground, preventing a player from really developing agility or other physical benefits. Improvements in agility and quick feet are possible only in the early years of training. After that, important changes, or adaptations, are necessary, such as introducing MxS and power training. Unless you employ strength periodization, your athletes will reach a plateau. However, it is not too late to apply periodization of strength methodology, where MxS is an important component.

3. Assuming that speed ladder exercises improve agility is a misconception because agility improves only as a result of fast and dynamic changes of direction, improving strength training, particularly maximum strength (MxS). Only MxS increases the force of push-off by recruiting a higher number of muscle fibers, by decreasing the duration of foot contact on the ground, and by increasing the thickness of the myosin.

4. For maximum benefit in the development of agility, use high-velocity speed and sideways diagonal movement, back and forth, at acute angles, 2-4 meters away from the median line of the exercise.

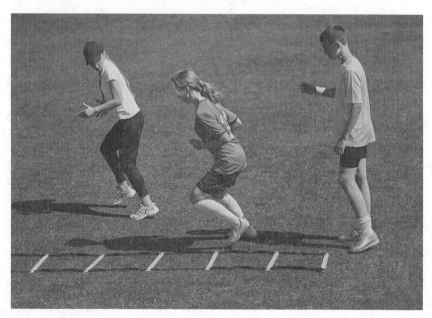

Figure 7.6 An example of a speed ladder.

During sprinting, the top sprinters apply a force 4–5 times their body weight against the ground (Churchill et al 2015; Dorn et al 2012; Monte et al 2020; Pandy et al 2021). But in speed ladder drills, the applied force is very low. Rather, specific sprinting speed, with maximum velocity, increases the speed of a player. Maximum speed is achieved by two athletic actions:

1. applying big force against the ground to increase propulsion force, to project the athlete forward/upward, and
2. maintaining a short duration of ground contact (which is directly dependent on MxS).

However, this is a good exercise for children U15–U17, mostly for developing foot and ankle musculature which is beneficial for your players as an injury-prevention strategy.

Lateral speed with elastic bands. In soccer, quick lateral moves are used during both defensive and offensive tactical actions. Lateral speed exercise is intended to improve the strength of the legs in order to move faster laterally. To accomplish this, an elastic band is placed above both knees with force applied against the band. The leading leg initiates the lateral motion while the trailing, or push-off, leg exerts the propulsion force against the ground to move laterally.

However, using this exercise in soccer training ultimately ignores the roles and activities of the legs. During lateral action in a soccer game, the lead leg does not encounter any resistance; it moves through the air. To move sideways, the trailing leg has the determinant role. This leg is the engine of lateral moves since it has to push sideways against the ground to overcome gravity and the athlete's own body weight.

In other words, when performing a lateral walk with a band, the person is loading the wrong leg and consequently there are no real training benefits. If you want to increase the force of the trailing leg, then you must increase the strength of the triple extensors.

Sled pull/push and parachute drag (figure 7.8). The idea behind pushing or pulling a sled is that it will help to develop speed. This exercise might be acceptable during general conditioning at the beginning of your annual training plan, but it is totally inefficient during the last part of the preparatory phase and during league games, when the scope of training is to develop and maintain the quality of speed, power, and agility.

The sled pull does not affect speed development because of the duration of the ground contact. For top players, the duration of ground contact is around 120 milliseconds (Charlie Francis, Canadian sprinting coach, and Bompa personal notes), but these exercises often have the athletes dragging the sled for far too long (300-600 m/s) which is not conducive to the development of speed and agility.

Parachute drag is also promoted as beneficial for speed training. It is claimed that having a player drag a parachute behind them will increase leg force and thereby improve their speed.

You know that sprinters in track are the fastest athletes on Earth. Have you ever watched how sprinters train? If so, you have certainly noticed they never use a parachute pull. This exercise is not conducive to increasing speed for one very important reason: the chute moves behind the player as they are running, creating instability and hesitation. Under these conditions, the player is trying to stabilize the body first, before pushing off, prolonging the foot contact, and any increase in the duration of foot contact on the ground means slowing the speed.

Of course, it looks spectacular, and it is fun to drag a parachute around, but the effect is far from what the ads claim. Instead, use maximum speed methodology (90-100 %), MxS, and power training.

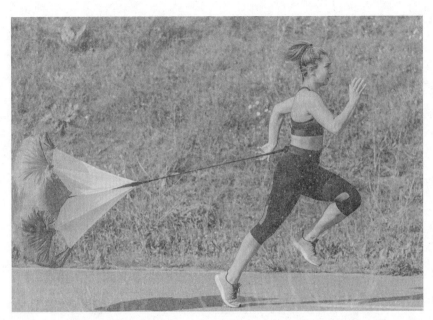

Figure 7.7 Example of a parachute drag. Note the arms' drive action that initiates the running action.

Fast running on the spot. Some internet enthusiasts claim that this drill increases speed. It does not. Increased velocity is achieved by improving force, not by more rapid leg movement (Weyand et al, 2010; Clark and Weyand, 2014; Seitz et al, 2014). Leg frequency relies on the intermuscular coordination: the coordination of the leg muscles to move the legs up and down with high frequency but low height.

Faster running speed is achieved as a result of applying greater force against the ground by the calf muscles, gastrocnemius and soleus, pushing forcefully and quickly against the force of gravity, not by more rapid but low leg actions (Weyand et al, 2000; Seitz et al, 2014; Pandy et al, 2021). If you want to improve your speed, increase your force application against the ground.

Exercises: Traditions vs. Science

Quite often the selection of exercises for fitness training for soccer has been based on tradition rather than the information from scientific study and methodological literature. Sometimes, track and field exercises are borrowed by soccer professionals, particularly from sprinting and jumping events, but since the early 2000s, the market has been invaded by commercial trends and its gadgets, of which many exercises and methods are completely ineffectual in soccer-specific training.

The opposite of this trendy (and ineffective) methodology is scientific and methodological studies in physiology of exercise, biomechanics, and electromyography (EMG), and this is what coaches should use to select the most effective exercises for their players.

The following discussion is intended to help you to increase your training's effectiveness, and to organize an efficient training program for your players:

• Legs are the determinant limbs in soccer. In order to achieve your athletic goals, legs have to be fast and agile, and neither is possible without specific strength training. Having weak feet and legs is like having a flat tire). **If you want to run faster, improve your legs' strength.**

• Figure 7.8 illustrates the prime movers for sprinting and high-velocity running: gastrocnemius and soleus, hamstrings, gluteus maximus, iliopsoas, and quadriceps. The low back muscles (lumbar), abdominals, and latissimus dorsi (used during the arm drive to pull the elbow backwards) are ancillary muscles. In other words, leg muscles are the actual prime movers.

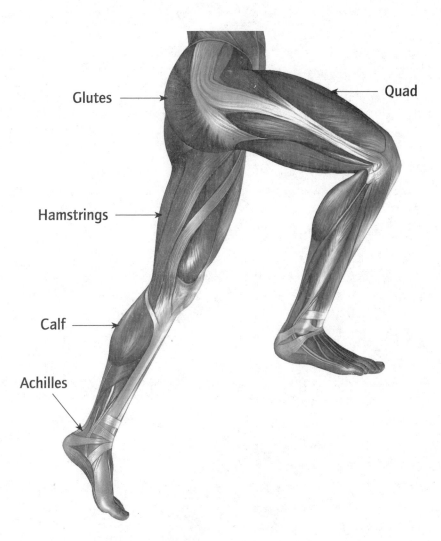

Glutes

Quad

Hamstrings

Calf

Achilles

Figure 7.8 The prime movers used in fast running. Note the complete push-off of the left leg performed by the gastrocnemius muscle.

Gastrocnemius: The King of Sprinting Speed

In order to target the prime movers of the leg (mostly the gastrocnemius and soleus muscles), squats, half squats, or step-ups (with a barbell on the shoulders) are often suggested. This approach is wrongly influenced by weightlifting and powerlifting. During the squat exercise, the most involved joints are the knee extensors (rectus femoris muscles), while the ankles are just partially active. In other words, the most important muscle used during running and agility, the gastrocnemius, is not efficiently targeted in squatting exercises. To effectively target the gastrocnemius, you have to use a calf press (at the leg press machine).

As shown in figure 7.9, gastrocnemius contributes 51 percent of the force necessary to achieve maximum speed in running and jumping performance, or maximum quickness in agility actions, while the rectus femoris contributes only 18 percent (Enoka, 2015). Therefore, to efficiently train the muscles needed for maximum speed, running, and agility, use the calf press.

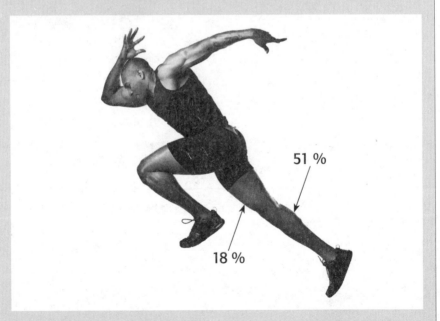

Figure 7.9 The percentage of contribution of the calf muscles during the propulsion phase in sprinting; gastrocnemius provides 51% while the quadriceps only provide 18% (Enoka, 2015).

Have you ever wondered why gastrocnemius is such a powerful muscle? The answer is that it has the highest number of muscle fibers, 1,120,000, and 1,934 innervation numbers that can be recruited to generate the highest force, speed, and agility (Enoka, 2015).How about the quadriceps? It has only 22,000 muscle fibers and 5 innervations numbers (Enoka, 2015)! Gastrocnemius has a determinant contribution to speed, agility, and jumping actions. The most effective exercises to strengthen gastrocnemius are calf presses and toe raises. Also remember that ground reaction force for gastrocnemius is 940.75 N, or 95.8 kg/221.2 lb (Richards et al, 2013). Ground reaction refers to the force applied against the ground by an athlete during sprinting or other athletic actions. The higher the force, the higher the ground reaction, and as a result, the higher the velocity.

Table 7.2 The difference between gastrocnemius and quadriceps muscles

Muscle	Gastrocnemius	Quadriceps
Number of muscle fibers	1,120,000	1,934
Number of innervation numbers	22,000	5

Data adapted from Enoka, 2015.

- This information should make you seriously question why great performance benefits are expected from training the quadriceps muscle (via squats exercises) when it has such a low number of muscle fibers, and thus a lower force production. Suggestion: replace squats with leg press and calf press.
- Soccer professionals should also consider the following research findings. When horizontal power was compared between sprinters and soccer players, the latter scored only half of sprinters' force: 15.7 Watts vs 7.9–11.9 Watts (Colyer et al, 2018). Clearly such a discrepancy in a sport where speed can have a determinant role in the outcome of the game proves that training methodology in soccer, specifically regarding strength, power, speed, and agility be carefully examined and improved. Contemporary training in soccer is a litany of quick fixes, instead of the physiological training it should be.
- As for the strength-training program, you may rarely see exercises being used to strengthen the hamstrings. Remember, fast running is the result of the contractions of gastrocnemius and soleus but also of the work

performed by hamstrings (mostly during the recovery phase of the running step). Rapidity in running also means fast contraction of hamstrings during the recovery phase of the running step. Weak hamstrings may impair your athletes' maximum speed because the knee flexion of the recovery phase is slow. In the case of agility movements, a weak hamstring means a slower deceleration action since hamstrings are highly activated during deceleration.

To train players to be fast and agile, use maximum strength (MxS) methodology to train your players' gastrocnemius, the main engine of speed and agility. This means using the calf press and leg press more often than doing squats.

As a strength and fitness professional you should be very careful about incorporating those exercises that are ultimately ineffectual and are not training sport-specific movements and skills. Instead train for maximum physiological adaptation. Finally, be very cautious about big lifts, including deep squats, snatches, and heavy-load powerlifts. Do not expose your players, particularly the young ones, to exercises with a high risk of injuries. Nowadays, there are strength-training machines that are better and safer than weightlifting and that can better target prime movers.

The Force-Velocity Relationship and Its Effects on Sprinting Speed for Soccer

Many aspects of the role of strength on the improvement of speed have been discussed previously. The aim of this section is to share with you more scientific information regarding the relationships between force and velocity and their benefits to the development of speed and agility. The following information is intended to demonstrate that without strong legs, the achievement of high speed and quickness is impossible. In doing so, we emphasize that

- high speed and agility are impossible to reach without first improving strength, and
- strength, particularly the MxS, is the source of maximum speed, take-offs, and agility.

The following comments (at times repeated to ensure higher retention) are based on the scientific and methodological studies that are so essential to consider when attempting to increase speed and agility in your soccer:

- Gastrocnemius (and not the quadriceps) is the major contributor to the development of speed, agility, and quickness while soleus is mostly active during the early part of the propulsion phase, having some contribution in all parts of the running step (Dorn et al, 2012). The stronger the gastrocnemius, the higher its contribution to speed and agility (Weyand et al, 2000; Colyer et al, 2018; Ferris and Hawkins, 2020; Pandy et al, 2021). Gastrocnemius is the prime mover for power, speed, and agility!
- Faster top running speed is achieved when greater force is applied against the ground, not by higher leg frequency (Weyand et al, 2000; Clark and Wayand, 2014; Udofa et al, 2017) such as fast running on the spot (figure 7.9). Fast running on the spot does improve coordination of leg muscles but does not have any effect on the developing speed.
- An increase in leg strength has a positive transfer to sprinting (Seitz et al, 2014; Clark and Weyand, 2014; Udofa et al, 2017; Schmidtbleicher, 2019; Pandy et al, 2021). Players exposed to MxS have stronger calf muscles. They can also generate the fastest speed because they can recruit a higher number of muscles fibers during the action.

- Faster runners generate higher speeds because they hit the ground with more force (Weyand et al, 2000; Udofa et al, 2017; Ferris and Hawkins, 2019; Pandy et al 2021). Therefore, S&C trainers should always remember that the force of propulsion (push-off) determines sprinting speed. In fact, even stride length is directly influenced by leg propulsion force. Modern soccer training seems to lack strength training, specifically MxS, and consequently S&C coaches should review their programs to be sure that they are incorporating the appropriate soccer-specific drills that will training propulsion force.

- At maximum velocity, sprinters can produce twice as much horizontal power as compared to soccer players: 15.7–17.9 Watts/kg vs. 7.9–11.9 Watts/kg. Why? Since most sprinters follow an organized strength training plan, they have twice as much power capabilities than soccer players (Colyer et al, 2018). Training to achieve high velocity is already part of many sports, but not soccer. However, as mentioned previously, strength and particularly MxS training will improve maximum velocity, making soccer players much faster.

- High level of sprinting speed can play an important tactical role by creating fast breaks, quick changes of direction, and by quickly altering the rhythm of the game.

- During high-velocity sprinting the vertical ground reaction can reach five times the athlete's body weight (Udofa et al, 2017). The higher the ground reaction, the faster the athlete. However, once again, in soccer, force is the answer to many aspects of training for increasing speed, agility, and jumping capabilities. Regretfully, some parts of contemporary training are far from what we consider strength/MxS training. Additional reading, however, will assist S&C instructors improve and apply the most recent information available in professional books.

- As speed increases from walking to sprinting (e.g., 2 m/s to 7 m/s), the force produced by gastrocnemius has the determinant role of reaching maximum velocity in running (Weyand et al, 2000; Hemner et al, 2010; Weyand et al, 2010; Schache, 2014; Ferris and Hawkins, 2020; Pandy et al, 2021). Therefore, exercises that are not specifically training gastrocnemius are a waste of time and energy. Maximum strength (MxS) methodology, if properly applied, will assist your players in improving maximum speed and agility.

- Calf press and leg press are the most efficient exercises for the development of calf muscles, the powerhouse of speed and agility actions, whereas squats are far from being a very effective exercise for the development of specific strength. These are the two very distinctive exercises that allow you to specifically target the development of the gastrocnemius and soleus.
- The propulsion phase of the running step (i.e., the push-off) is the most important element necessary to achieve maximum speed (Hemner et al, 2010; Udofa et al, 2017; Pandy et al, 2021). Use leg and calf press exercises to strengthen the muscles responsible for generating force during the propulsion phase: gastrocnemius and soleus. Effectiveness in training is higher when you plan a lower number of exercises with a higher number of sets per muscle group.
- **Ground reaction** (GR). When players initiate a move such as (walking, running, jumping), they apply a force against the ground to perform the action. At the same time the ground reacts with an equal force in the opposite direction (Newton's third law of motion: action–reaction). Depending on the angle of the force applied, GR can be vertical or horizontal. When runners push backward against the ground, they benefit from GR, which pushes the player forward (thrust reaction force), much like the recoil of a spring. The higher the backward force, the higher the forward thrust.
  - » When the player applies force against the ground, they can benefit from the GR by increasing the impulse during the push-off, pushing the player forward. In all athletic moves horizontal impulses are applied in every contact with the ground.
  - » The force of GR is of similar magnitude to the impulse of the propulsion phase (i.e., the force of the push-off of the running step). If a runner applies force against the ground, the GR is equal to that force, achieving a corresponding velocity. If a runner desires to generate superior velocity, he must apply higher force. Higher force always elicits a higher reaction and, as a result, improved speed performance.
- Duration of the foot contact on the ground is physiological element that determines high-velocity running: the shorter the duration of foot contact on the ground, the faster the player. Let us take an example: a sprinter covers 100 meters in 50 strides, with a duration of foot contact on the

ground of 120 milliseconds. His opponent does the same, but with a shorter duration of contact phase, 110 milliseconds. Who is the faster athlete? The athlete whose duration of contact phase is shorter.

- To decrease the duration of foot contact on the ground, a player must increase the maximum strength (MxS) of the calf muscles. Weak calf muscles result in an increased duration of foot contact on the ground which delays the time to start the propulsion phase, and, as such, decreases velocity.
- All ground-based moves are a function of the force applied against the ground. Quick horizontal acceleration, rapid, short sprints, and agility moves determine success in soccer.
- High sprinting speed is achieved by pushing and not by pulling (e.g., overspeed training, pulling a sled). During pulling of a resistive action, the duration of the contact phase increases visibly, and the speed decreases.

Sprinting Speed and the Role of the Achilles Tendon

Top soccer players are always among the best in technical finesse, tactical proficiency, and physical potential. They rarely miss the opportunity to hone all the qualities necessary to excel. They are also concerned with maintaining every small detail of the game at a high level. Among these details is the state and strength of the Achilles tendon.

Tendons have a very important property: they can store high mechanical and elastic energy that is released during running and agility drills. The thicker the tendon, the higher its elastic properties. Longer tendons, such as the Achilles tendon, have a longer arm of force and lever: a clear mechanical advantage during sprinting, jumping, and agility actions. We suggest players work to increase and maintain the thickness and flexibility of the Achilles tendon via MxS.

To best understand the role of the Achilles tendon during sprinting, jumping, and agility, you must compare it with the role of the string of a bow. During the stretch, the string stores elastic energy. When the string is released, the elastic energy is released, propelling the arrow forward. The higher the elastic energy (stretch of the string), the faster the arrow travels. If you have a strong arm, you can increase the stretch of the string, and as a result, the arrow will travel with an even higher velocity.

When gastrocnemius muscle contracts, it transmits mechanical force via the Achilles tendon to the bone to initiate a physical motion. Every time you want to display a higher force, you need a proportionally stronger Achilles tendon. As you work to increase muscle strength, you have to also create a specific training program to improve the strength of the Achilles tendon (please refer to the last part of this section).

The Achilles tendon can transmit the highest force of all tendons of the body: 4900 N/510 kg/1124 lb (Enoka, 2015). A weak Achilles tendon is an impediment to achieving high force and high velocity. If you want to generate high force to improve your speed and decrease during agility drills, you must increase the strength of gastrocnemius and Achilles tendon.

Any increase in ankle and Achilles tendon force results in decreasing the duration of contact phase of the running step (Udofa et al, 2017; Werkhausen et al, 2019). The shorter the duration of the contact phase, the higher the running velocity. You will never have a fast or agile player that has a longer duration of the contact phase.

Powerful muscles always have thicker cross-sectional areas than tendons. In fact, there is a direct correlation between elastic properties of a tendon and its thickness. A strong Achilles tendon also has a larger area of insertion (65 mm^2, Enoka, 2015). The stronger the tendon and the larger the insertion area, the better insurance there is against injuries. Always remember that high force is equal to high velocity.

A low level of strength will never produce fast players.

If the tendon is weak, the transmission of high mechanical force is also weak. Therefore, weak tendons are least effective and can be exposed to discomfort and even injuries. Some sprinters, particularly those with low strength, have higher incidents of injuries at the place of insertion of the Achilles tendon on the bone calcaneus.

The force displayed by muscles depends not only on the activity of cross bridges (refer to the sliding filament of myosin with actines) but also on the elasticity of the tendons.

Please note that it is essential to continually work on expanding the range of motion and flexibility of the Achilles tendon (stretching it, bringing the toe as close to the tibialis bone as possible). Low elasticity and reduced range of motion may result in tears or even breakage of this tendon during high mechanical stress.

Take time to strengthen your athletes' Achilles tendons! The most effective exercises are calf press, short and fast sprinting, plyometrics, bounding exercises, rope jumps, hill raise with weight in your hands or on your shoulders, running on stairs, and reactive jumps.

Reaction and Movement Time Training

Many fast, quick movements in soccer are not possible without also relying on reaction and movement time. To initiate a quick action or reaction, the sensory organs must first be aroused, followed by a nerve impulse to the brain, and then a muscle contraction before an overt movement can begin. These processes involve time, and together they constitute reaction time.

Figure 7.10 outlines reaction time components:

1. The appearance of a stimulus at the receptor level (visual, auditory, tactile)
2. The propagation of the stimulus to the central nervous system (afferent or sensory transmission)
3. The decision-making process in the central nervous system (CNS)
4. The transmission of the signal from the CNS through nervous pathways to the muscle (efferent or motor transmission)
5. The stimulation of the muscle to contract and perform the movement (well-trained muscles react and contract faster)

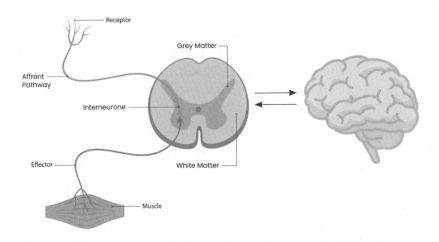

Figure 7.10 The paths of reaction time from receptors to the muscles, the effectors (Bompa, 2006).

Training Simple Reaction Time

Goalies, defenders, and offensive players must respond quickly to numerous stimuli throughout a game. Players are sometimes faced with a single stimulus, such as reacting to a ball passing by or how an opponent is positioned during the game. This describes a simple reaction time situation. A simple reaction is a conscious response to a previously known stimulus performed unexpectedly.

- Choice reaction time. During practice or competition, players encounter several stimuli (i.e., game-specific conditions) that they must react to. For example, a forward must find an open space and react to opponents' actions and initiate tactical maneuvers. The act of the forward choosing from several possibilities is called a choice reaction. A goalkeeper goes through similar processes when defending a shot on goal. In this case, the goalkeeper must choose from stimulus-response alternatives such as speed, direction, and spin of the ball before responding appropriately.

Obviously, a player's reaction speed is fastest when only one stimulus is involved. When the number of possible options increases, there is a gradual increase in the choice reaction time required to respond to any one stimulus. Thus, these situations provide us with information about the different decision-making processes in the nervous system of the brain.

- Reflex reaction time and speed refers to rapid responses, be they voluntary or involuntary, to stimuli that involve little or no conscious control. A knee-jerk reaction is a great example of this. When a defender encounters a sudden move made by an opponent, this player's muscles and limbs adjust automatically to the force with an equal amount of resistance. These automatic responses can be modified via conscious perceptions of sensory information or based on experience accumulated from learned actions during training and games. Over time, these learned responses may become automatic.

Training Methods for Developing Reaction and Movement Time

The concept of reaction time exists and has been used in training by some coaches for many years. It is not a novelty, but we brought it back in our discussion particularly for improving goalie training. Fast reaction time represents a great advantage for most players, often with dramatic effects for the goalies. Although the ability to react quickly is inherited, at least to some degree, others can be improved with proper training.

Reaction time to a visual stimulus, such as a ball in motion, is shorter for trained individuals (0.15–0.20 seconds) than for untrained individuals (0.25–0.35 seconds). This time is even shorter for elite players (Canadian Hockey Association,1995 and 2016). Several other sources indicate that reaction time to an auditory stimulus, such as the yell of a teammate, is slightly shorter at 0.17–0.27 seconds for untrained individuals and 0.05–0.07 seconds for world-class players. Tonnessen et al (2013) reported that top male athletes react extremely quickly to the sound of the starting gun: 0.142 seconds for male athletes and 0.153 for female athletes.

The improvement of reaction time depends largely on how well the players understand the drills and exercises, as well as how motivated and focused they are to perform the specific tasks. If a player's concentration is directed toward the drill to be performed, rather than on how fast they hear the signal, reaction speed will be much faster. Reaction time is also faster if the player slightly pre-contracts the muscles required to perform the action (i.e., contracts the relevant muscles before the stimulus).

Drills for reaction and movement time can be performed at the beginning of a training session when players are fresh. Occasionally, however, these drills should be performed under conditions of fatigue to prepare players for similar conditions that arise during the latter stages of a game. Use your imagination to create new and interesting drills to prevent monotony and boredom in training.

Audiovisual Training

The audiovisual training method is based on the relationship between reaction time and the ability to distinguish minor lapses, or micro intervals, of one tenth of a second. It is assumed that those who can perceive small time differences between various repetitions will develop good reaction times.

A simple but effective training method involves repetitions in which the player reacts to both auditory and visual signals, such as a whistle, hand clapping, or any stimulating sound. Consider the following examples:

Drill 1: The player backpedals toward the coach. At the coach's signal, the player turns to face the coach, who uses an arm to indicate the direction in which the player must move as quickly as possible.

Drill 2: The player runs backward toward the coach. At the coach's signal, the player turns to face the coach, who throws a ball—in a different direction each time—that the player must quickly control.

Drill 3: The coach stands to one side of the goal. The player backpedals or shuffles sideways away from the coach. At the sound of the whistle, the coach passes a ball in a given direction, forcing the player to change direction quickly, control the ball, and shoot on goal. The player can also be given the intermediate task of controlling the ball while running around a cone before shooting to score.

Drill 4: The player performs a reaction drill from lying on the field in various positions. At the coach's signal, the player stands up as quickly as possible and performs the action or task indicated previously by the coach. Alternatively, have two players push each other with equal resistance. At the coach's signal, they must perform a predetermined technical or reaction drill. Combine this exercise with various ball actions, such as slaloming between cones, zigzagging, and so on.

Drill 5: The player moves in a specified direction. At the coach's signal, the player performs a reaction or technical task. If shooting or attacking is involved, the coach will indicate at which part of the goal or court to shoot or spike.

Reaction Ball Training

Besides the traditional drills used to train movement time for goalies (or any other player), players can also use a reaction ball to improve reactivity by performing the following exercises:

Drill 1: Players throw the ball against the wall and catch it as quickly as possible.

Drill 2: Same as drill 1, but players kick or hit the ball in a predetermined direction.

Drill 3: Players stand 3-4 m (around 10 ft) away from a wall. They throw the ball against the floor and wall and try to catch it as quickly as it rebounds off the wall.

Drill 4: Same as drill 3, but players use a foot to stop and control the ball.

Drill 5: Throw the ball onto the floor and have two to four players battle to gain control of the ball with their arms or legs.

Drill 6: Throw the ball against the wall, let it bounce, and have two to four players battle to gain control of the ball and immediately attempt to throw it at a given target.

Drill 7: Interrupt the player's concentration (e.g., look at the ceiling), then quickly throw the ball in a given direction. Have the player gain control of the ball and throw or shoot at a predetermined goal.

Because of its bumpy shape, a reaction ball thrown against the floor or wall always bounces in an unpredictable direction, thus challenging players to quickly react. Reaction balls are quite effective but rarely used in soccer training. Many years ago, I introduced it to ice hockey.

Conclusions

How can your players play a fast game if they have not been trained to be fast?

High sprinting speed is the most desirable physical ability in soccer, particularly during offensive tactical actions, when maximum sprinting speed is determinant. Train your players carefully, make them strong and fast. Please disregard some traditions that might not serve you well and organize the best training sessions possible.

There are far too many gimmicks in soccer training. Most are promoted as being effective when often the reality is exactly the opposite. Some leg exercises, running on the spot or with little push-off action, are a waste of time. Some of them may look interesting, but they do not improve any aspects of your players' abilities.

The determinant element for improving speed is not the design of the drill but rather its physiology, intensity, and maximum speed. Many speed and agility drills are made with the same speed and intensity, changing only the design of the drill. Design is good for variety, but please remember the drills must be performed with high speed. Doing them at low/medium speed results in little to no benefit.

The traditional fitness programs for soccer must be improved upon. The exercises that make up the program must be soccer-specific if they are to train players' speed, agility, and quickness. By incorporating the exercises suggested as part of MxS training, you are guaranteed to develop a successful training program for your players.

CHAPTER 8
TRANSFORMING MXS INTO AGILITY AND FLEXIBILITY TRAINING

KEY POINTS

- Agility Training
- Deceleration-Acceleration: The Key to Agility and Quickness
- Guidelines for Agility Training
- Periodization of Agility
- Program Design
- Flexibility Training
- Developing Flexibility

Since most information presented in this book is in condensed form, agility and flexibility are presented together in this chapter.

Agility Training

Agility training trains the ability to quickly and suddenly change direction by moving the feet fast and with high rhythm, and to swiftly accelerate and decelerate to achieve a tactical action. Good timing, high-frequency footwork, and quick reactions are also intrinsic elements of agility. It is one of the most important physical qualities of soccer. Yet, agility is a combined quality and does not exist independently, but rather it directly depends on the level of other fitness actions, such as power, speed, frequency, and reactivity.

Basketball or handball players are good examples of agility as they exemplify high-frequency footwork. When watching these players, one can see how quickly they move their legs on defense. To effectively guard their goal or basket, the players' legs are constantly moving swiftly and in different directions.

Developing quickness and agility directly depends on improving leg strength, particularly that of the calf muscles (gastrocnemius, soleus, and tibialis anterior) and thigh muscles (quadriceps). Yet, some training specialists still view agility as evolving from speed. However, they should remember that speed itself directly depends on a player's leg MxS and power, and that only a powerful player can be a fast soccer player. This is also true about agility: Only powerful players can be agile. Please remember that nobody can be fast, be agile, or have quick feet before developing strength.

Deceleration-Acceleration: The Determinant Element of Agility

High-level agility, rapid changes of directions during the game, can be attained in two phases:

- **Deceleration**, or to first slow down almost to a stop, results from the eccentric loading (lengthening) of the quadriceps muscles.
- **Acceleration**. The elastic energy stored in the muscles during deceleration is then used during acceleration, when players begin to run quickly again. Rapid change of direction relies on two main muscle groups: gastrocnemius and soleus (calf muscles) and the quadriceps (thigh muscles). To quickly accelerate with the gastrocnemius and soleus (dominant muscle groups for this action) have to contract concentrically during the acceleration phase. This is why the ability to decelerate and accelerate quickly does heavily rely on the ability of these muscles to contract powerfully, both eccentrically and concentrically.

The deceleration–acceleration coupling will never be fast unless MxS and power are properly trained. Agility actions requiring quick feet to rely on leg power. In order to defend against offensive players, you need strong legs. Also, to elude a defender, forward players must rely on two elements:

1. *The technique of the first step* has to be performed quickly, depending on how quickly the player drives the opposite arm. If a player initiates a forward step with the left leg, the quickness of the step depends on how

fast the player moves the right arm forward. The arms and legs always move in perfect, alternating synchronicity and coordination, in the following sequence:

a.   the arm drive, and

b.   leg reaction (to the arm motion). Both actions are performed in just a fraction of a second.

2.   *The force applied against the ground*, the propulsion phase, has to be very powerful, and dynamic. It is applied eccentrically (ankle dorsi flexion, and knee and hip extension). The force of the propulsion phase depends on the amount of force load during the eccentric contraction. The higher the eccentric load, the more dynamic the propulsion is.

Agility ladder: Have you noticed that it is used to train agility from childhood to maturity? And yet we rarely question how effective this exercise is for most players. Although teenagers can improve agility from repeating various exercises on an agility ladder, how about mature players? Do they gain anything from these exercises repeated already for more than 10 years? We really doubt it!

Did you ever time the duration of the agility drills/courses you use for your players? You might be surprised to learn that the duration is 4–8 seconds! It is rarely longer than 10 seconds! What does this mean? What is the training effect of an agility routine for a player where the duration of a game is 60–90 minutes? Don't you feel you may have to revise your training methodology, eliminate the gimmicks of the day, and use energy systems training methodology instead?

Guidelines for Agility Training

As a very important physical quality in soccer, agility has its own training methodology which includes the following elements.

Intensity

For best results, agility and quickness drills have to be performed at a very high intensity: 90–100%. If intensity is lower, as witnessed in contemporary agility training, you certainly are training something, but not agility!

Since elevated intensity relies on the neuromuscular system and the quality of agility exercises is very much dependent on the neural responses and reactivity of this system, this type of training is often referred to as neuromuscular training. The potential of the central nervous system (CNS) to send powerful, fast, and high-frequency impulses to the fast-twitch (FT) muscle fibers involved in performing agility exercises directly influences the discharge rate of FT fibers. Do you want to improve your players' agility and quickness? Perform agility drills with good technique and high intensity.

Duration

For best, game-specific, position-specific adaptation, the duration of agility exercises, drills, and courses have to be organized as per the specifics of energy systems:

- 5–12 seconds for exercises taxing the phosphagen/alactic energy system
- 20–30 seconds or higher, for drills taxing glycolytic/lactic acid energy system
- Over 1-2 minutes for the aerobic system. Players cannot be expected to play at a high rhythm for long if the agility drills do not tax, at least partially, the aerobic energy system.
- Rest interval between repetitions has to allow at least partial recovery, 1-2 minutes, especially for the drills taxing the alactic system. A longer time of 3 minutes is suggested for drills taxing the glycolytic/lactic acid energy system, since this type of training is very demanding physiologically. Finally,

for drills taxing the aerobic system, the rest interval has to be relatively shorter at 2 minutes, since these types of drills are not as taxing on the glycolytic system.

- Total time for agility training per training session, including rest intervals, can be as high as 20-30 minutes.

It is the coach's responsibility to gauge the progression and intensity according to players' positions, backgrounds, and physical potential.

Duration of Foot Contact

To best benefit from the effect of the stretch reflex, foot contact with the ground should always be on the ball of the feet. This is called *light feet* and is characterized by springy actions generated by the muscle's elasticity. Hard landing, on the other hand, is called *heavy feet, since landing on the ground occurs* on the soles of the foot. Any lengthening of the duration of the contact phase on the ground results in a significantly slower, sloppy movement. Therefore, players emphasizing light feet must perform agility exercises quickly, with a short contact phase, and maximize the elasticity of the muscles.

Listen to How the Step Sounds

Listening to the sound of players' steps provides important feedback regarding the quality of the exercise. Observing how your player executed an agility drill is as important as listening to players performing an agility exercise, paying particular attention to the ground contact. Noisy, clapping sounds are an indication that your players' feet are landing on the sole, rather than on the ball. Therefore, the players' movements reduce the effectiveness of performing fast and quick agility drills. A *quieter*, fluid, and springy agility action and soft ground contact reveals your players' levels of MxS and power.

Note: Please also keep in mind that clapping or noisy feet, especially towards the end of a workout, may also be an indication that players are experiencing neuromuscular fatigue.

Observe the Height of the Step

The height of the player's steps should remain as low as possible so the player can get the foot back in contact with the ground quickly for another push-off. For the fastest agility actions, players should consider stepping below ankle height and as quickly as possible between the two points of the agility step: the push-off and landing phase. The dynamic elements of movement requiring speed and quickness occur in the push-off or propulsion phase. The more frequently a player pushes against the ground, the faster that player moves.

Detecting Player Fatigue

Fatigue is the result of many elements of soccer training. However, every type of power, speed, and agility training used in soccer affects the state of the neuromuscular system, the neural reactivity of the fast-twitch muscle fibers. Therefore, the negative effects of fatigue also diminish the quickness of contract.

Fatigue, particularly that of the CNS, directly deteriorates the technique of all skills performed by players, including performing agility drills effectively. If players look sloppy, the foot contact is prolonged and noisy, and if the heel touches the ground, it is a clear demonstration that the neuromuscular system is fatigued or even exhausted. Under these conditions, coaches should stop the drill, provide a longer rest interval (>4 minutes), or even conclude the workout.

Periodization of Agility

As a well-organized coach, you certainly know that planning and periodization agility training can guarantee that your coaching activities will result in the best training adaptations and performance improvements.

The periodization models (figure 8.1) may be used as a guideline for you to create your specific agility training model. Please note that the level of strength development, particularly MxS, is essential for any substantial increase in agility. The adage that nobody can be agile before being strong has never been truer.

Preparatory		League games
No games	Exhibition games	Maintain power, agility, quickness, specific endurance
Adaptation	MxS, power, agility, quickness, speed endurance	

Figure 8.1 Periodization of agility and quickness during an annual plan.

Following a well-deserved vacation, players return to the club ready to prepare themselves for the next league games. The new training plan starts with an adaptation (A) phase, where they are exposed to a progressive training: technical, tactical, strength, power, speed, agility, flexibility, and specific endurance.

During the second part of the preparatory phase, players are also involved in exhibition games. This program represents a testing assessment for the coach, who, based on his or her conclusions, can make the necessary changes prior to the start of the league games. Finally, during the league games all the fitness elements of training have to be maintained. Why? What is not trained will detrain.

Planning Agility Training in a Workout

High-intensity training should occur immediately after the warm-up, when the CNS is still fresh, well-rested, and able to respond quickly to various stimuli.

However, if the goal of a specific training session is to train quickness and reaction time under the conditions of fatigue, agility exercises should be trained towards the end of the session. Although fatigue interferes with the reactivity of the CNS, players can adapt progressively to a high level of fatigue and still perform fast and quick movements.

Considering this training objective, drills must remain short (5–10 seconds) and must be performed as quickly as possible. This approach must be employed if players are expected to be sharp, fast, and explosive as at the beginning of the game.

Designing an Agility Course

During the preparatory phase, fitness instructors and coaches should design agility courses, not just agility drills, for each energy system starting from the MxS phase on. Agility courses should be based on the energy systems. Agility courses can be designed in any area, pitch, park, or gym, using any kind of equipment available to you: benches, low hurdles, markers to make a slalom activity, jumps over various equipment, back paddle, etc. Your imagination is the limit. This type of training should be mostly planned for the lactic acid system, or as a short exercise for the aerobic system (2–5 minutes).

Program Design for Agility

Most training methods for the development of agility involve acceleration, deceleration, and changes of direction. For best game-specific adaptation, agility actions can be trained with or without the ball. At times, you can use the ball with agility courses, since this training option may be more challenging and fun.

Please note the terminology regarding agility actions: the term *drill* is intended for shorter duration activities, taxing the phosphagen (alactic) energy system, whereas a *course* is of a longer duration, taxing the glycolytic (lactic acid) system.

Table 8.1 can be used as a guideline to design your own programs as per the specifics of facility availability and individual player's potential. Please note that instead of distance to run you may also use the time equivalent of that duration. In this case please do:

- 5–10 seconds for agility drills, taxing the alactic energy system
- 30–60 seconds for agility courses, taxing the glycolytic system
- 3–5 minutes agility course, taxing the aerobic energy systems.

For additional enjoyment and technical challenge, you can also use the ball to control it throughout the agility course.

Table 8.1 Training guidelines for agility drills and courses

From of training	Distance (m)	Number of repetitions	Rest interval (min)	Number of training sessions per week
Without the ball				
Acceleration-deceleration	10-30	6-10	3-4	1-2
Acceleration-deceleration-acceleration	20-40 for each segment	4-8	3-4	2
With the ball				
Acceleration	10-30	4-6	2	2-3
Deceleration	10-20	4-6	2	2
Stop and go	10-20	4-8	2	2-3
Acceleration/ direction changes	10-30	4-8	2	2-3
Agility course				
Lactic acid system	200-400	2-3	3-4	1-2
Aerobic system	600-800	1-2	2-3	1

Contemporary training in soccer is full of agility drills, often to the point of overdoing them, but some instructors miss a very important training element: that good development of agility directly depends on the level of development of MxS. Therefore, while a lot of time is dedicated to the improvement of agility, some instructors neglect *the source of agility: MxS*. If MxS is overlooked, any gains in agility during the early part of fitness training will *plateau*!

As already mentioned, agility courses can also be designed as per the specifics of energy systems: lactic acid and short aerobic. You may be surprised how much enjoyment players may experience, particularly if they use the ball. Agility courses are fun but also challenging physiologically.

Flexibility Training: A Very Condensed Form

Flexibility, often called joint mobility, refers to the range of motion around a joint, or the amplitude of a joint to facilitate specific motions with ease. Flexibility training also plays an essential role in your strategy to prevent injuries. As an important training concept, S&C trainers must be mindful that flexibility of a joint must be greater than the degree of amplitude of a joint during the game. Please consider this simple game situation: as a ball is coming to a player's chest, the player must attempt to control it by lifting a leg up to that height. If flexibility training was inappropriate, the player lacks the flexibility to lift his leg and control the ball.

Flexibility training must be part of every training session, immediately after the warm-up, when muscles are warm and ready for 10-15 minutes of stretching. A well-designed program that successfully develops flexibility must be long term, beginning from childhood, when muscles are easier to stretch; done at the same time as technical training; and maintained the entire time the player is playing soccer.

Flexibility training in soccer involves repetitive movements, often through a limited range of motion, such as longer strides or attempting to control the ball at head level. This can lead to muscle tightness and possibly muscle strain and tears. A careful and progressive increase in flexibility will comfortably allow the player to stretch the muscles, relieving muscle tightness and helping prevent injury.

Flexibility training in soccer should specifically address the ankle, hips, groin, and adductor muscles, which are active when sliding and tackling. Like other soccer attributes, flexibility must be effectively trained to allow the muscles to adapt and enhance the quality of play (Hebert and Gabriel, 2002; Ingraham, 2003; Stoddard 2016). This is why flexibility has to be multifaceted and include all training methods, particularly dynamic stretching prior to workouts and games. It must be an ongoing training concern for all soccer players, although girls have better flexibility than boys, especially after puberty, when boys grow stronger muscles. Stronger muscles are always more difficult to stretch. From puberty on, the trend of sex differences continues, although girls seem to reach a plateau (Alaranta et al., 1994; Kohl and Cook, 2013) that will not affect their quality of game. From this age on the main concern are not the girls but rather the boys.

Many exercises used in soccer to improve flexibility are far from effective. Nor do they properly target the correct anatomy of a soccer player. Please refer to the following exercises (figures 8.2-8.4) which specifically develop the flexibility of those major muscles and joints used in soccer. You may also consider placing them in your injury-prevention program.

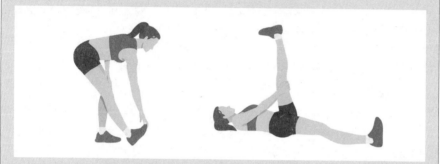

Figure 8.2 Suggested for stretching the hamstrings, a sensitive group of muscles for all players.

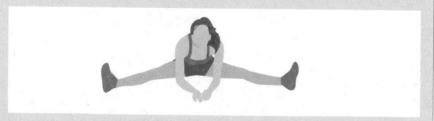

Figure 8.3 An effective stretch exercise to increase flexibility of the adductor muscles.

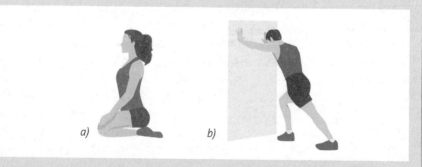

Figure 8.4 Exercises for the ankles, one of the most neglected joints in soccer. (a) plantar flexion; (b) dorsi flexion.

Training Methodology

Training methodology for the development of flexibility uses three methods: 1) static (stretching and holding a position at an acute angle for 5-10 seconds; 2) dynamic (stretching muscles to their limit and actively bobbing the muscles to reach their limits of motion); and 3) proprioceptive neuromuscular facilitation (PNF), such as stretching the muscles to their limits, holding that position for 4 or 5 seconds, then stretching again to the limit. This latter method can also be trained with a partner; when one athlete reaches the limit of flexibility, the partner can apply pressure to extend the degree of flexion or extension beyond that limit.

There seems to be a geographical preference regarding the methodology of flexibility. From 1970-1990, most coaches and athletes from North America preferred static stretching while in Europe, the preference was dynamic flexibility, particularly in the traditional sports of track and field and gymnastics. Recently, however, dynamic flexibility has gained some recognition in the North American, supported by many scientific publications (Kumar and Chakrabarty, 2010; Blackhurst et al., 2015; Stoddard, 2016).

Overall flexibility is a necessity, but, as also mentioned, ankle, knee, hip, and groin flexibility is a must. Most instructors have a decent knowledge regarding exercises for flexibility. To best serve your players in your desire to prevent muscle and ligament problems, you have to make sure that you are addressing the following muscles and tendons: Achilles tendon, leg adductor muscles, hamstrings, quadriceps, and trunk flexion-extension and rotation.

Selected Comments About Other Training Options in Soccer

In their quest to offer variety in training, some coaches appeal to other options, such as:

- Sand training. The theory is that it develops power and endurance. However, since sand does not offer firm support, ground reaction is prolonged, far from developing power, and ineffective. Similar experiments were also used in playing in snow in a reduced terrain. Though they offer fun, variety, and resilience, these options cannot replace good, high-intensity sprinting speed and agility.

- Training accessories. There is an abundance of training accessories: running over low hurdles, running over rings, slalom running around various markers. All the exercises are good for children and as added variety for mature players, but physiological benefits for top players are limited. As you already know, without physiological improvements there are no athletic gains, no matter what kind of accessories you may use.

Conclusion

Speed and agility are highly regarded abilities in soccer. Coincidentally, both of them are directly dependent on the level of development of MxS. Please remember the following:

- MxS has a determinant role in the continuous development of agility.
- If you spend some time observing the training program of a top soccer club, you will be surprised to find out that many parts of the program are not of high quality. Many drills are just a simulation of high-intensity training.
- Without using high intensity during agility drills, your work as a trainer is not soccer specific, and, therefore, ineffective. On the other hand, if you maintain the same type of intensity, your players will reach an undesirable physiological plateau.
- Organize your agility training based on the physiological principles of energy systems.
- Agility must be trained not only to tax the phosphagen (alactic) energy system but also the glycolytic system (lactic acid), so essential during the attacking–counterattacking strategies of your team. If the glycolytic energy system is not well trained, the continuous, strenuous attacks–counterattacks and high rhythms of the game will be a physiological impossibility.
- Flexibility in soccer is of a modest quality and inadequately trained. Regretfully, stretching is not exercised methodically, as it is in gymnastics, swimming, and other sports. In most cases, hip flexibility is repeated during drills for agility, where lifting the knees to horizontal is regarded as flexibility. Flexibility has to be used not only to properly elongate some muscles but also for the post-game, post-workout recovery and regeneration.

CHAPTER 9
DEVELOPING SOCCER-SPECIFIC ENDURANCE

KEY POINTS

- Factors Affecting Endurance
- Fatigue and Recovery
- Guidelines for Endurance Training
- Developing Specific Endurance
- Developing Game-Specific Endurance
- Developing Position-Specific Endurance

If you are considering the contribution of energy systems in soccer (alactic 15%, lactic acid 15%, aerobic 70%), the contribution of the oxidative (aerobic) system throughout the game is dominant, significant for a player's final performance. Endurance refers to the capacity to perform longer-duration work at a given resistance. Fatigue is the main factor limiting the endurance capabilities of soccer players, in general, and game-specific endurance in particular. Players are said to have good endurance capacity when they do not fatigue easily, or when they can cope with and continue to train or play in a state of fatigue.

Along with strength training, the weakest link in soccer is endurance training. When players fatigue fast and recover slowly following training and games, it is a clear indication of a low level of endurance.

Factors Affecting Endurance

As a physical quality, aerobic endurance is essential in many aspects of the soccer game, particularly at the end of each of the two halves, when players encounter the highest level of fatigue. When it comes to endurance and soccer, it is important to remember that:

- endurance and aerobic capacity depend on long-duration methods used during training;
- energy reserves (energy available to the player) depend on energy expenditure during training and a player's nutrition plan;
- energy expenditure depends on the rhythm and duration of the game and training sessions;
- perseverance is a psychological quality, tested by the game or type of training; and
- fatigue is a multi-factor issue and depends on all of the above.

It is important to be aware of several factors that may help or hinder the development of endurance:

Central nervous system: When a player is exposed to endurance training, the central nervous system (CNS), his organs and systems, adapts to the specifics of the training demand, its volume and intensity, ultimately increasing its working capacity. Fatigue, which often impairs training and play capacity, occurs at the CNS level. Therefore, a decrease in the working capacity of the CNS is a major cause of fatigue. The struggle against fatigue is a battle of the bodily systems and the player's willpower to maintain a high working capacity.

Willpower: Player's willpower is an important ingredient they can use in their quest to improve endurance. Every time a player is forced to perform under conditions of fatigue he must rely on his willpower. Mental fortitude and strong willpower are in higher demand as intensity increase during training. To maintain the required training intensity, players have to also appeal to the nervous centers to continue working at the same level or higher, particularly at the end of a game. Finally, to maximize their endurance capacity, players have to appeal to both training methodology but also to overcome the weaknesses that often accompany fatigue.

Aerobic capacity: The body's capacity to produce energy in the presence of oxygen (O2), determines a player's endurance potential. A player's aerobic capacity is often limited by the ability to transport O2 to the working muscles. As a result, improving the delivery of O2 to working muscles should be part of every program designed to improve aerobic endurance. A good aerobic capacity facilitates faster recovery between training sessions and after games. Furthermore, a rapid recovery represents a sign of good aerobic endurance that also allows players to reduce their rest intervals and perform work at higher intensities.

Anaerobic capacity: Performing a tactical drill with high intensity depends on how much energy is supplied by the anaerobic system, the energy produced in the absence of oxygen (O2). Players' anaerobic capacity is affected by CNS processes, which facilitate work under fatigue or exhaustion. If players improve their aerobic capacities, their anaerobic capacities will also improve. As a result, players will be able to work efficiently for longer periods of time before the levels of blood lactate increase and affects further training. Finally, players with high aerobic capacities recover faster from the fatigue incurred during the game but can also maintain a high rhythm of the game at the end of each half.

Fatigue and Recovery: A Summary

This topic has been left for the end of this discussion simply because it is an essential element in soccer to always remember, a sort of conclusion of this chapter.

Fatigue is regarded as a state of tiredness; lack of energy; reduction of physical, technical and tactical capacity; and the decreased ability to play at a high rhythm or a quality game. Often, the end result of a soccer game depends on the level of fatigue players have encountered and how fatigue has been managed by the players of the two teams. A player that experiences a high level of fatigue is often inhibited to perform maximally. Players undergo the highest level of fatigue in different parts of the game, usually during the early part of the second period and, more evidently, at the end of each half (Moh et al, 2004; Oliveira Goulart et al, 2022; Dambroz et al, 2022).

In a systematic review of female soccer players, Oliveira Goulart et al (2022) found that post-game sprinting and jumping abilities decreased by 1%, while Dambroz et al (2022) reported that fundamental parts of the game, such as passing, dribbling, game tactics, and sprinting, were visibly affected by fatigue. Negative effects of mental fatigue, in the form of players' synchronization capacity, accuracy of decision making, accuracy of passing, and maximum velocity, have also been reported by Kunrath et al (2020). It is not a coincidence, but most non-contact injuries also occur in the latter part of the game, when players' fatigue is also the highest (Dupont et al, 2018).

Recovery, in simple terms, refers to the strategies you can take to counteract or reduce the effects of fatigue, including the risk of injuries, via dietary, psychological, and physiotherapy techniques, with the goal being to quickly return to the pre-fatigue state (Marques-Jimenez et al, 2017; Oliveira Goulart et al, 2022).

Among the rational methods of recovery, we can suggest undergoing a cool-down, including lots of stretching of the highly taxed muscle groups (calf and thigh muscles). Not surprisingly most players from the English Premier League dedicate about 40% of their time to stretching (Dadebo et al, 2004; Dupont et al, 2018). However, Herbert and Gabriel (2002) reported that stretching has not been proven clinically. However, Octavian Popescu, MD (1958), proposed that stretching is essential to speeding up the process of recovery for the simple reason that it elongates the muscles. Popescu claims that when a muscle reaches the longest anatomical length, it facilitates the best biological exchanges and faster elimination of residues from the muscles, such as lactic acid.

Dupont et al (2018) proposed that the process of post-game recovery should start immediately via:

- hydration (water and salt): 500–700mg of salt per liter of water,
- a drink of cherry juice and chocolate milk to restore glycogen,
- a cold bath, 12–15°C for 10–20 minutes,
- a meal high in carbohydrates with a high glycemic index, and
- a good night's sleep.

Guidelines for Endurance Training

If you decide to improve resilience, the game- and position-specific endurance methodology, your players must develop the ability to overcome fatigue to adapt to all training demands of the game. Successful adaptation is reflected in improved endurance, which is demonstrated during training (performing endurance activities without difficulty during highly demanding training sessions, games, and testing. S&C coaches must also strive to develop all three types of endurance (alactic, lactic, and aerobic), according to the specifics of the game of soccer and the position they play. The development of endurance depends on the volume and intensity of training planned by the coach.

Alactic and Lactic Endurance Training Guidelines

Most of the methods used for developing alactic (phosphagen) and lactic (glycolytic) endurance involve high-intensity activity. The following guidelines may be used to better understand the specifics of lactic and alactic endurance:

- Training intensity may range from sub maximum to maximum levels. Although a variation of intensities is used during training, intensities around 90 to 95% of maximum should be emphasized for improving alactic endurance (Bangsbo, 2014; Bompa and Buzzichelli, 2019).
- The same authors suggest that the duration of work may last 5–90 seconds, depending on the energy system the player is targeting—less than 12 seconds for the alactic system and 20–90 seconds for the lactic acid system.
- The RI following an activity of high intensity must be long enough to replenish the O2 debt. Recuperation is a function of the intensity and duration of work and may take between 2–7 minutes. Plan the longest rest interval so that the accumulated lactic acid will have sufficient time to oxidize; players can then start the next set almost fully recovered (Dolci et al, 2020).
- Activity during RIs must be light and relaxing (e.g., jogging or low-intensity technical skills, such as precision passing) to facilitate recovery and energy replenishment. Total rest (i.e., lying down) is not advisable because this causes a drop in the excitability of the nervous system.

- Since work designed to develop alactic capacity tends to be very intense, the number of repetitions must remain at low (3–4) to medium (5–6), which supports training at high intensity.
- If the goal of training is to improve lactic endurance, the number of repetitions is higher, often 9–12.

Aerobic Endurance Training Guidelines

Physiologically speaking the benefit of aerobic training increases more effectively when you use lower intensity but longer duration/distance. However, this concept is a rarity in soccer since the contemporary fitness training is mostly composed of short agility-type drills that are taxing the phosphagen (alactic) energy system. Therefore, soccer players rarely train the aerobic system, and, consequently are not well adapted to it. It's no surprise then that soccer players have difficulty maintaining aerobic activity for extended periods and suffer the effects of fatigue relatively quickly. On the other hand, players with good aerobic endurance can maintain continuous endurance activity, better tolerate fatigue, and recover faster following training.

When you train aerobic endurance, please consider the following methodological guidelines:

- **Intensity:** For best adaptation to aerobic training, intensity has to be below 70% of maximum aerobic velocity, at an approximate heart rate of 140–164 beats per minute (bpm). If the heart rate per minute is not above 130 bpm, training benefit will have an insignificant effect on the improvement of aerobic endurance. Therefore, as a guideline for maximum aerobic training, U17-U19 players may consider a heart rate of around 200 bpm, with girls often registering a higher rate of around 6-8 bpm.
- **Duration** of aerobic training can vary between 45-60 minutes, or longer, of steady-state training. Plan this type of training during the early preparatory phase; in the second part, you can use repetition training methodology of 60–90 seconds, with or without the ball. This type of training results in the adaptation and improvement of lactic-acid tolerance training players encounter during the game. Longer repetitions and tactical drills, of 2-5 minutes are also needed to improve game-specific aerobic endurance via specific technical and tactical drills.

- **Rest intervals** between repetitions should fall between 90 seconds to 3-5 minutes. Longer rests can cause the capillaries (the blood vessels that connect arteries with veins) to constrict, thereby restricting blood flow for the first few minutes of work. The heart rate method can also be useful for calculating an appropriate RI. Usually when the heart rate drops to 120 bpm, work can resume without difficulty (Bompa and Haff, 2009).
- **Activity during RI** is normally of low intensity to facilitate natural biological recuperation. Walking and jogging are familiar activities for well-trained athletes, but easy passing or ball control exercises of low intensity can also be performed during RI.

Training Methods for Developing Specific Endurance

Soccer players can develop endurance by using a variety of methods that produce very specific physiological and performance responses. When developing a training plan, the coach must determine the type of endurance that the plan will target because methods of developing endurance are vastly different in their implementation and physiological outcomes. For example, traditional methods to develop the aerobic system call for continuous training performed at a variety of intensities ranging from 60-90% of maximal heart rate (Bompa and Haff, 2009; Bangsbo, 2014). The use of high-intensity interval training has been reported to improve anaerobic endurance, thus increasing the training options available to the coach and player (Bloomfield et al, 2007; Bangsbo, 2014; Perroni et al, 2019). Conversely, short duration dominant training methods, including the contemporary training drills, appear to decrease aerobic capacity, which would ultimately impede the player's capacity to perform at a high rhythm of the game. Coaches and their players must be aware of the different methods used to develop both aerobic and anaerobic endurance and which kind of endurance is more soccer or position specific.

Note: The aerobic system in soccer is grossly neglected simply because of the influence of commercialism in training and, at times, a superficial knowledge in sports science, physiology of soccer, and training methodology. Therefore, some fitness trainers are taxing just the alactic system via some agility-like drills (e.g., slalom, speed ladder, runs in various directions). Let us remind you that the alactic energy system, prevalent in contemporary training for soccer, represents only 15% of the energy used during the game. What happened to aerobic training that ensured fuel for 70% of the game?

When and how is aerobic endurance trained in the era of ineffective exercises and training methodology? Now you know why the rhythm of the game cannot be maintained for the entire duration of the game.

Aerobic Training Methods

The most commonly used aerobic methods used in soccer are uniform (steady state) and tempo training. Let us briefly discuss these two methods:

Uniform (Steady-State) Method

A continuous, high volume of work is typical in the uniform, or steady-state, training method. The uniform method is used during the early part (2-4 weeks) of the preparatory phase. If some players have a longer preparatory phase the uniform training method can be prolonged by 1-2 weeks. For top players with shorter preparatory phase, uniform training can be replaced with tempo training (chapter 7). The technique of running uses a comfortable stride length, performed with ease and uniformity.

The appropriate intensity for a given steady-state training session can be calculated using the heart rate method; the rate should be between 130–164 beats per minute (bpm), always keeping in mind individual differences. The main training goal is to improve players' aerobic capacities. Although the uniform training method is not very effective for top players, for children under 17 years of age, it is essential to build an aerobic base, develop the lungs' capacity, and organize an injury-prevention training, such as the adaptation type, to strengthen the leg muscles, ligaments, and tendons.

Repetition and Interval Training Method

Since both methods have many similarities, they are presented together. The base for aerobic and anaerobic endurance must be built during the early part of the preparatory phase and maintained during the league games.

Repetition training is a more formal method:

- Set the distance of repetition training (e.g., 20 m, 40 m or longer).
- Set a specific intensity as a percentage of maximum velocity (e.g., 70%).
- Set the duration of the rest interval (e.g., 2 min).

Interval training is less formal than repetition training and a more fluid and flexible method. Often during rest intervals, players can perform activities with the ball. An example of interval training using non-stop, tactical activities with the ball includes:

- Transition drill: from offense to defense (2 min)
- Transition drill: from offence to defense, defense to offense, and repeat once more, ending with a counterattack (repeat 2–3 times, 3–4 min)
- As above but with a higher number of non-stop repetitions of offence-defense (5 –10 min)

These suggestions might be a surprise to some S&C coaches who have been relying too heavily on current training trends and have not been using game-specific endurance training.

Repetition Method

Considering the specifics of soccer (time motion analysis) and the contribution of each energy system during the game, the jogging drills that abound in contemporary soccer training do not meet the needs of the game-specific endurance. Since jogging does not accurately reflect the intensity of the game, and since it does little for the specific aerobic adaptation of the organs and related functions of most players you may consider other training methods such as repetition and interval training, which more closely reflects the dynamic nature, pace, and rhythm of soccer.

The varied endurance training methodology has a cumulative benefit for your players, so it has to be applied according to your players' aerobic capacity, facilities, game schedule, and so on. Please remember that a single repetition of one minute tempo/tactical drill relies almost entirely on the anaerobic system, but several repetitions covering the same distance provide, cumulatively, more specific anaerobic–aerobic benefits. During repetition and interval training, lactic acid is always building up, demonstrating that the anaerobic energy system can no longer supply the necessary fuel (glycogen), so the body must tap the aerobic system for additional energy.

Repetition training is a relatively simple method in which players have to repeat specific distances, from 20–150 m or longer, alternating with a set rest interval. Start with the longer distances and, as players adapt to this work and league games approach, progressively decrease the distance but increase the intensity of each repetition. The suggested intensity is distance-related: higher intensity, 80% for short repetitions and 50-60% for longer repetitions. Longer, game-specific repetitions place a stronger emphasis on the aerobic component of the game, resulting in improving game-specific endurance. Alternatively, shorter and higher intensity repetitions/tactical drills are more game-specific because the speed resembles game speed conditions. Higher number of repetitions at the desired pace are quite challenging, resulting not only in improved game-specific endurance, but also challenge the mind, but help players to strengthen their willpower. The total number of repetitions, 5->8, is distance-related (more repetitions for shorter distances). The volume of work may be 20–30 minutes, with a rest interval (RI) of 3–5 minutes, depending on the distance and intensity of the repetition.

Training plans should recognize the technical, tactical, and physical characteristics of soccer and enhance the physiological and motor skills required during a game (table 9.1).

Coaches can create their own plans or models by first making a list of the activities or actions players perform during a game. Of course, position-specific details must always be kept in mind, since only then will players be trained according to the specific physiological demands and physical qualities necessary to excel at their positions.

The repetition method offers you varied possibilities such as:

- Sprint, pivot, stride, side shuffle, bending run, stop and go, compensation activities (e.g., jogging/rest)
- Acceleration–deceleration, deep, acute angle of slalom run, cruise, backpedal, compensation jog between activities
- Stride, side shuffle, change of direction, pivot, compensation jog between activities
- Sprint, stride, stop and go, backpedal, forward sprint, compensation jog between activities
- Acute angle slalom run, stop and go, bending run, acceleration–deceleration, leap over simple obstacles, compensation jog
- Simple obstacle course, jump over obstacles (e.g., cone, bench), change of direction, jog, acceleration–deceleration, compensation jog, rest
- Simple tumbling, series of leaps, side shuffling, crossovers, spike jumps (players hold a medicine ball in both hands and throw the ball over a volleyball net), changes of direction (5-10 in different directions), jogging, low-impact plyometrics, overhead and sideways medicine ball throws, compensation jogging
- Backpedaling, side rolls, dives with quick recovery to the feet, push-ups, acceleration–deceleration (5-10 m in various directions), jogging, simple plyometrics, medicine ball throws, compensation jogging
- Skipping rope, overhead and sideways medicine ball throws, reactive jumps, jogging, changes of direction, acceleration–deceleration, side shuffling, dives, jogging, backpedaling, step-ups, compensation jogging

Table 9.1 Suggested guidelines for repetition and interval training

Type of activity	Distance (m)	Intensity % of maximum	Rest interval between repetitions (min)
Sprinting	10-40	90-100	2-3
Striding	30-50	70	2
Cruising	20-40	50	1-2
Bending run/cuts	10-30	80-100	2-3
Acceleration-deceleration	10-20	80-100	2-3
Acute angles slalom/changes of direction	20-30	80-90	2
Stop and go	10-20	80-100	2
Side shuffle	10-20	70-100	2
Forward run and backpedal	10-20	70-90	2-3
Tempo running	50-150	60-80	2-5 (higher intensities require longer RI)
Simple obstacle course	50-100	60-75	2-3
Tactical drills: Employ IT methodology	As per the energy system you want to tax: 45 seconds-5 minutes	60-90	3

Data adapted from Bompa, 2006; Bompa and Buzzicelli, 2011.

Note: If the suggested rest interval is not long enough to allow the players to recover to your desired level, it may be extended by 1–2 minutes.

Interval Training

Since early 1920s interval training (IT) has been used as a very successful method to develop aerobic and anaerobic endurance. IT involves the repeated performance of short to long bouts of exercise usually performed at or above the lactate threshold, interspersed with periods of low-intensity exercise or complete rest. Although interval training is not a new training method (it was made popular in the 1930s by the German mid-distance runner Rudolf Harbig), an increased interest in the concept has stimulated a great deal of research in the area of sport science. This scientific literature has revealed many physiological reasons why interval training should be an integral part of the annual training plan for soccer players. Interval training can be subdivided into two broad categories: aerobic and anaerobic intervals.

Aerobic Interval Training

IT for the development of the aerobic energy system involves intensities that are at or slightly above the lactate threshold (lactic acid build-up in the blood stream is at a higher rate than it can be removed). At that point, the player's motivation is highly challenged, as often happens during the game, particularly when the game is of constant intensity or at a high rhythm.

Aerobic IT has also been termed *threshold training or pace or tempo training*. Pace or tempo training can be performed continuously or intermittently. For example, in a continuous pace or tempo training session, the player would maintain a steady pace at or slightly above the lactate threshold for the duration of the exercise bout.

Aerobic intervals can also be set by prescribing a heart rate range for a predetermined duration (Bangsbo, 2014; Dambroze et al, 2022). The rest interval can be preset to specifically target the development of the aerobic system. For example, a player may perform eight sets of aerobic intervals that last five minutes and are separated by one minute of low-intensity active recovery. The intensity for this type of interval would be 80–85% of maximal heart rate or some percentage of the lactate threshold heart rate.

Regardless of the method used, aerobic intervals can stimulate significant physiological adaptations when performed two times a week for up to four weeks prior to the start of the league games. Because of the large amount of physiological and psychological stress that can be generated by aerobic interval training, the coach should decide on a specific rest interval (table 9.1).

Anaerobic Interval Training

Anaerobic interval training for endurance athletes has recently received a large amount of attention in scientific literature. In this type of interval training, the work duration is very short (<2 min), and the intensity is maximal. As an example, anaerobic interval training may use bouts of 4-10 sets of 15-30 seconds of all-out intensity, interspersed with 45 seconds to 1 minute of recovery. This type of training has been shown to significantly increase VO2max and anaerobic endurance and stimulates many physiological adaptations that improve performance in as little as two weeks (Laursen and Jenkins, 2002; Bompa and Haff, 2009). These types of training sessions are usually very intense and require the use of recovery methods and appropriate program variations to avoid exhaustion. It is likely that this type of training can be very effective when performed one or two times per week and integrated into the training plan.

Developing Game-Specific Endurance

For maximum benefit and to achieve complete body adaptations, aerobic and anaerobic training must follow a game- and position-specific method. As a result, several of the methods and variations presented in this chapter should be used to achieve the best physiological adaptation and psychological benefits, such as maximum concentration, willpower, perseverance, and aggressiveness.

Aerobic training for soccer is quite complex in itself and can be used with or without the ball from the early preparatory phase on. In addition, you should use game- and position-specific aerobic endurance methods along with technical and tactical and strength and power training, applying similar methods as suggested in previous sections. To create your team's training plan to develop and maintain all three energy systems used in soccer, the following specific drills can be designed to enhance a given energy system:

- High-intensity drills below 12 seconds tax the alactic energy system.
- Intensive drills of 20–90 seconds tap the lactic acid system.
- Continuous drills of medium or medium-high intensity of 2–5 minutes or longer (up to 10 minutes) can be used to develop or maintain the aerobic needs of your players. For maximum tactical anaerobic effectiveness, create tactical drills with the ball that might be part of your game strategy for the following game. Use repetition training methodology to train your players to adapt and play with a high rhythm of the game for its entire duration. To avoid high-intensity exhaustion (alactic-lactic), workouts can also be organized to alternate energy systems, on separate days to facilitate recovery and regeneration (table 9.2).

Table 9.2 A suggested week (microcycle) of training with one game per week

Day	1	2	3	4	5	6	7
Activity	Game	Recovery techniques	Training	Off	Training	Training	Game
Energy systems	All	Aerobic	Alactic/ lactic		Lactic/ aerobic	Alactic/ lactic (short # of repetitions)	All
Training demand	High	Low	High		High	Low	High
Training objective	Apply game tactics and objectives	Recovery: light activities with/ without ball, physio-therapy	T/TA drills	Recovery, regeneration, specific nutrition, physio-therapy	T/TA drills based on game plan set for the next game	TA drills as per the tactical plan set for the next game	Apply game tactics and objec-tives

Legend: T= Technical; TA=Tactical

Note: Please observe the alterations of energy systems and training demand. Two other examples of micocycles with one and two game per week are illustrated in chapter 10, tables 10.5 and 10.6.

Developing Position-Specific Endurance and Soccer Abilities

As already known, each position on a soccer team has its own physiological characteristics that must be trained in order to train your players. So to accommodate the specifics of each position on your team, training programs must incorporate exercises and drills that mimic players' positions and the specific physiological requirements as per the dominant energy systems. Along with the specific energy system training, most players also need to be exposed to training programs for developing sprinting speed, agility, and quickness (such as simple tumbling, varied and continuous jumps, dives and rolls, reaction and movement time, exercises that train game-specific actions and reactions, and so on).

Table 9.3 Position-specific abilities required for a soccer team

Position	Energy systems	Dominant elements of strength	Dominant physical abilities
Goalie	Alactic: 100%	MxS Power Reactive power	Power, jump power Reaction time Movement time
Sweeper	Alactic: 30% Lactic: 30% Aerobic: 40%	MxS Power Reactive power	Starting and jump power Reaction and movement time Maximum acceleration-deceleration Quick turns
Fullback	Alactic: 20% Lactic: 30% Aerobic: 50%	Power Power endurance Agility	Starting power Maximum acceleration-deceleration Quick turns and changes of direction Reaction and movement time
Midfielders	Alactic: 10% Lactic: 20% Aerobic: 70%	Power endurance	Power endurance Speed endurance Reaction and movement time Acceleration-deceleration

Position	Energy systems	Dominant elements of strength	Dominant physical abilities
Strikers	Alactic: 20% Lactic: 20% Aerobic: 60%	MxS Reactive power Power endurance	Power Starting power, jump power Maximum acceleration-deceleration Reaction and movement time Quick turns
Wings	Alactic: 20% Lactic: 30% Aerobic:70%	Power endurance	Power endurance Speed endurance Maximum acceleration-deceleration

Compiled based on information from: Ekblom, 1986; Bangsbo 2006; Bompa, 2006; Bloomfield et al, 2007; Thorpe et al, 2017; Perroni et al, 2019; Dolci et al, 2020; Bompa and Sarandan, 2023.

Comments Regarding Some Training Drills

Certain aspects of contemporary fitness training without the ball include a multitude of drills using gadgets and training accessories. Although some drills are useful and fun, most of them contradict the energy systems, and physiology, of soccer. From injury prevention to soccer-specific endurance training, some aspects of contemporary fitness training for soccer are, at best, of modest quality.

- Despite knowing that aerobic endurance represents 70% of the energy necessary during a game, drills for specific endurance are missing from some training plans.
- Some training drills are intended for the development of speed. Yet the velocity players use during a drill looks more like jogging or, at best, of medium intensity and speed! To improve speed, use drills of maximum velocity.
- If anaerobic, aerobic endurance, and high sprinting speed are not trained, coaches cannot expect their players to be fast and resilient and able to sustain the high rhythm of a game.

Conclusion

The development of aerobic, anaerobic, and game-specific endurance is extremely important for achieving overall endurance training. During the transition from aerobic to anaerobic and game-specific endurance, it is essential to maintain aerobic endurance. High-intensity training, a hallmark of the league games, may not produce the desired results unless a solid foundation of endurance is established during the preparatory phase.

Specific endurance, for the latter part of the preparatory phase and throughout the league games, can be best achieved via drills with the ball but of typical duration for the anaerobic and aerobic drills.

Revise your fitness training program to leave behind all the ineffective exercises and methods and create your own energy systems-specific drills based on the specifics of the physiology of soccer.

Some aspects of contemporary fitness training rarely plan training sessions for the development or maintenance of game-specific endurance. Why? For the simple reason that some instructors are relative novices in the area of fitness training for soccer while commercialism is interested in the commercial aspects of soccer.

Finally, the notion of fitness training at a high level, including game-specific endurance, is missing from their repertoire.

PART IV
PLANNING AND MODELING IN SOCCER

Effective coaches are good planners! In the last part of this book, select plans for soccer are proposed for your consideration. Why? Because planning equals efficiency. Although you are using your own system of planning, a quick perusal of the following plans might trigger your interest to evaluate and compare what you do with what we propose.

These plans are just guidelines. They are not rigid items but rather a training instrument to be altered as needed by the specifics of training and game schedule. Additionally, we also included several models of training for you to use or adapt according to your needs.

CHAPTER 10
SIMPLE PLANNING AND MODELING IN SOCCER

KEY POINTS

- The Integrated Game Models
- Simple Models for Simulation Training
- Model Training Plans
- Modeling the Annual Plan: League Games
- Modeling the Microcycle
- Modeling Weekend Tournaments

To some, planning and modeling seem very similar. However, for our purposes, a plan is an outline of a training program. A model, on the other hand, represents a plan that is tried and tested, and can be reused in the future.

The concept of modeling in sport science has its foundations in mathematical methods of modeling. Since the inception of sport science, there have been a wide array of scholarly publications, particularly after the 1990s and 2000s. However, in both theoretical development and practical application of modeling, we are still in the state of infancy.

As an important training concept, modeling has the scope to simulate and create in training technical and tactical models that should be reproduced during the game. These strategies prepare players for different game situations and social environments. In sport training sciences, modeling has been applied in many areas, including:

- statistics and game analysis (Avalos et al, 2003),
- modeling the coaching process (Cushion, 2007),
- computer simulation for tapering (Luc et al, 2009),
- as an organizational tool for professional sports (Cyrenne, 2009),

- for modeling sports tournaments (Cattelan et al, 2012),
- imagery in sports psychology (Law, Post, and McCullagh, 2017),
- as a model for performance excellence in sport psychology (Aoyagi et al, 2018), and
- computational models applied to learning science, sport psychology, biomechanics, and game analysis.

Modeling is also used to mimic training technical, tactical elements, and physical and psychological skills that will be used in the tactical plan you create for the next game.

As you make the game plan, you should also consider how your players' abilities can be integrated into the team's philosophy and how individual players fit into the overall game plan.

Finally, you should plan specific training sessions to ensure a game-specific adaptation that should improve game effectiveness and result in a better game and a superior performance.

The Integrated Game Plans and Models

Planning and periodizing training are essential parts of a coach's activity before he or she starts training the team for the following league games. Obviously, a plan is just a flexible guideline to follow that must be adapted as per the specifics of the games and team's training status. This guideline is called the integrated game model, and is the cornerstone of a team's future training program for the entire duration of league games.

The integrated games plan begins first with setting the team's performance objectives; these should be challenging but also realistic and attainable. The team objectives set by the coach must include the qualities of the available players for each position, their technical and tactical and physical abilities, and, conversely, the main elements of the system of play to be used. The technical, tactical, and physical models consist of each individual player's game plan that is to be integrated into a model for the entire team. Finally, the physical demand model must evaluate players' fitness capabilities, whether they can adapt to the systems of play used by the opposing team, and must also consider their intensity capabilities and overall resilience.

An example of an integrated game plan and model includes the following steps:

- Performance objective
- For the entire team
- For each individual player
- Game model
- Formations and positions
- Between lines and groups
- Transitions from offence to defense, and defense to offense
- Tactical model
- Offensive model to be employed
  » Counterattacks
  » Positional attacks
  » Flexibility in adapting the model to the opposition's system of play
- Defensive system to be employed
  » Against fast breaks
  » Against positional attacks
  » In special game situations
- Technical model
- Skills necessary to apply the tactical model
  » Predominant skills used in offence and defense
- Model the physical demand of the game
- Your team's model
- The opposing team's model
- Model the game's environment
- Hostile audience
- Intimidating strategies
- Equipment, playing conditions, quality of the field
- Model the players' theoretical knowledge
- Team tactics
- Psychological skills required during the game
- Model the expected organization and conditions of the game to be played
- Time of the game
- Quality of officiating
- Monitoring and analysis
- Evaluate the game's model

- Analyze the players' application of technical, tactical, physical, and psychological models
- Positive and negative conclusions for the future
- Proposed changes for the future
- Conclude with realistic optimism for the future

The Environmental Model

Being aware of the environment in which your team will play helps you avoid negative surprises. A model for playing environment refers to:

- the circumstances under which the players play the game, such as equipment, time of the game, quality of officiating, and whether the players had a chance to work out on the field or in the gym before the official game, and
- the sociopsychological climate (how the spectators may affect team performance). Often, an unfavorable environment leads to high tension that disturbs psychological processes such as concentration, self-control, combativeness, perception, lucidity, reaction time, and decision-making process. A friendly audience could stimulate these traits, resulting in a better performance.

Steps for Developing an Integrated Model

Creating a game model follows these steps:

1. A thorough analysis (*analysis phase*) of the effectiveness of last season's training and game plan (i.e., how successfulthe team was), and
2. A thorough analysis of individual player achievements. Based on this analysis, training elements are retained or replaced with new concepts in all elements of training (technical, tactical, physical, psychological, and social).

In the next step, new qualitative elements (e.g., training volume and duration, number of repetitions) are introduced (*introduction phase*). The new game model is then tested (*testing phase*) in training and later in exhibition games. If not totally satisfied with the team's performance during the testing phase (*validation phase*), coaches still have an opportunity to make any necessary changes before the league games start, and to finalize the model (*finalization phase*) to be used in the upcoming competitive season (*application phase*).

The steps (phases) for developing a new game model for the next league games:

1. Analyze the past season.
2. Introduce new training elements.
3. Test the model.
4. Finalize the model.
5. Apply the model in exhibition/league games.

The best time to create a new model is during the transition (off-season) and the new preparatory (preseason) training phases, when the stresses of competition are absent. This is an ideal time for a comprehensive and critical analysis of the previous year's game model, including re-evaluating whether the objectives, tests, standards, and training parameters were set and accomplished adequately. Similarly, analyze how the player coped with training and game stressors, and find ways to improve this is the future. Then, objectively select the methods and means of training that will materialize in the new game model, eliminating those that were ineffective.

It is possible to make changes to the basic model during league according to the new team's performance. Alteration of the model is necessary if the team does not match performance expectations.

Model Training to Simulate Game Conditions

Simulation is a method intended to replicate fundamental elements of a competitive game, establish specific technical and tactical schemes, and standardize certain parts of the game plan with the ultimate goal of increasing the team's effectiveness. It is equally important that coaches evaluate, using individual tools, whether the simulation models translate well to game situations and whether players are effectively following the tactical model. For maximum effectiveness, each game model must be repeated during training so that it becomes a standard prototype, a pattern. Rehearse these models under game-specific conditions, including when players experience high levels of fatigue or even exhaustion. The following simulation model may be used:

- **Simulation of the teams' tactical plans** should consider placement on the field, player and ball movement during the game, offensive and defensive strategies, face-offs, and tactics after scoring. In other words, specific tactical elements are repeated frequently during practice to produce actions that are likely to be used in upcoming games or tournaments.

- **Simulation of the interaction between two or more players**, including the tactical role of the playmaker, tactical support given to teammates in scoring position, and tactical approach after a successful or unsuccessful offensive sequence. To achieve maximum benefits, this model must be repeated many times during training to make sure that players forming a specific line become familiar with each other's roles on offense and how to cover each other on defense.

- **Simulation of the game's technical demand** has to consider the technical and tactical roles and variations of offensive and defensive players. Defensive roles could often mean disruptions of the tactics used by the opposing team, while offensive refers to the use of effective technical and tactical skills and maneuvers or clever fakes to create an effective offensive drive. Allow adequate time during workouts to simulate and rehearse these specific skills.

- **Simulation of individual tactical actions**, such as a player's position within the structure of the team, and of the players that have special degree of tactical freedom within the team's game plan, both on offense and defense. These players, particularly on offense, must have tactical intelligence, be flexible tactically, and possess ingenuity and excellent fitness and resilience.

- **Simulation of the game's physical demands**. Having excellent fitness has to be based on the specifics of energy systems for soccer. Power, sprinting speed, agility, quickness, as well as game- and position-specific endurance are among the main attributes of a well-trained player. To develop all these physical qualities, your training program must start from the early preparatory phase as per the periodization concept. The effectiveness of soccer-specific fitness training can be even more efficient if these abilities are exercised as part of the complexity of tactical training with the ball.

- **Simulation of signs used to communicate specific tactical actions** must also be part of the team's tactical training. Create specific drills to simulate the signs you will use during the game. In many cases, communication among own players is the attributes of the playmaker, captain, or a midfield player. Once again, simulate the use of these signs during specific parts of the training session, particularly when you rehearse tactical maneuvers.

- **Simulation of the game environment** by duplicating adverse circumstances similar to the away game, such as hostile audience (noise), biased officiating, unfavorable playing conditions (deteriorated playing surface, wet field, unfamiliar goals or balls), playing at an unfamiliar time of day, etc.

Model Training Plans

Any training program can be modeled to coincide with the objectives of training, depending on what goals the coach's plan aims to achieve. Creating a model for a given training program, therefore, provides an advantage for the coach and players because a certain physical quality or skill can be developed according to the specifics of the game. The training model described here refers only to the training sessions, microcycles, and annual plans.

Model training and training plans are suggested for training sessions, microcycles (weekly training plans), and the entire year of training leading to the league games. It is very important that the coach model training for the microcycle, the best and easiest planning tool to work with. There are other options that the coach can select depending on the scope of training and abilities to develop.

The annual plan is mostly a guideline, simply suggesting the ability to train and its duration. Please also note that this plan refers to the preparatory phase only, the first two months of preparing for the league games.

Modeling Training Sessions

Training sessions are among the most practical and applied types of plans that can target specific objectives that are technical, tactical, or physical in nature. Successfully achieving your training goals directly depends on how the session is organized. Please avoid using the same type of training session with the same objectives and structure. In other words, attempt to avoid boredom! In addition, this will keep your players motivated and enthusiastic about improving their technical and tactical skills and physical potential. The following training session models and plans were designed with this in mind.

Model Training for Skill Acquisition

Technical proficiency, the enhancement and refinement of new skills, is essential for each and every player and can be achieved by following the following training structure:

1. Warm-up: 20 minutes running, calisthenics, and good overall stretching, particularly for the ankles, Achilles tendon, knees, and hip and groin muscles.
2. Technical and tactical drills that teach or refine a skill or improve the accuracy of passing and shooting: 60 minutes.

The benefits of this training model are not difficult to justify. Specific skill training should occur before the central nervous system (CNS) becomes fatigued, since it is a well-known fact that fatigue affects execution and retention of some skills. Therefore, drills for skill acquisition or accuracy should immediately follow the warm-up when players are still fresh. In addition, plan longer rest intervals to prevent fatigue and to facilitate maximum skill retention.

Do not plan skill acquisition for the end of a training session when the players are more likely to be fatigued.

1. Physical training (improve or maintain strength): 30 minutes.
2. Cool-down: 10–15 minutes. Stretch the limbs and muscles used in training, elongating the muscles to their anatomical length to facilitate the removal of metabolites from the system, including lactic acid.

Note: The proposed warm-up and cool-down should be applied to all the following models proposed.

Model Training for Skill Acquisition Under Conditions of Fatigue

Since fatigue is an undesirable condition during the game, you must take every action possible to improve players' capacity to tolerate fatigue and improve their skill acquisition under adverse physiological conditions, using the following training model:

1. Warm-up: 20 minutes.
2. Technical and tactical drills that tap the lactic acid and aerobic systems: 50 minutes.

3. Speed or power training using specific or nonspecific exercises and drills: 20 minutes.
4. Technical and tactical drills to improve accuracy of passing and shooting under conditions of fatigue: 20 minutes.
5. Cool-down: 15 minutes.

This structure will assist your players in adapting to high conditions of fatigue, improving skill retention when fatigue starts to set in, and improving tolerance of increased lactic acid for the rest of the game.

In order to achieve and even to enhance the above objectives, you may also plan some fitness training under the same physiological conditions.

Model Training for Speed and Power Development

Developing power, speed, quickness, and agility, is best done when players are rested, relaxed, and recovered from previously acquired fatigue. The following suggested training session structure can help you achieve these goals:

1. Warm-up: 20 minutes.
2. Specific or nonspecific drills and exercises to develop power, speed, and agility: 30–40 minutes.
3. Technical and tactical drills for skill automation: 45–60 minutes.
4. Cool-down: 15 minutes.

Model Training for Speed and Power Development Under the Condition of Fatigue

Soccer games are played fast, with a high, dynamic rhythm, that often can be adversely affected by fatigue. This is not the case during the early part of the game, but, obviously, poses visible technical, tactical, and physical problems when players are in a state of fatigue, especially during the late stages of a game.

As most technical and tactical errors are made late in the game when fatigue affects the accuracy of passing, shooting, and tactical thinking, the same situation occurs when players want to display game-specific moves dynamically with high speed and sharp agility. Once again, fatigue interferes with players' desire to perform technical and tactical maneuvers with the same intensity and dynamism.

Soccer games are won or lost at the end, when players are still expected to maintain the fast tempo of the game, quickness, powerful actions, consistency, and resilience. However, quick and powerful actions are affected by fatigue. Unless you organize a training structure that facilitates speed and power training under conditions of fatigue, do not expect miracles from your players in the final minutes. To overcome these potential barriers to performance and improve the team's performance in the later stages of the game, the following training model is proposed:

1. Warm-up: 20 minutes.
2. Technical and tactical drills of longer duration that tap the aerobic system and fatigue players: 60 minutes.
3. Speed and power drills performed under conditions of fatigue: 30 minutes.
4. Cool-down: 15 minutes.

Your goal is to organize 60 minutes of technical and tactical drills, with each drill being 30–60 seconds, typical for lactic acid (glycolytic) endurance training, that can be performed immediately after the warm-up. The scope of this part of training is to intentionally fatigue your players! This type of fatigue is similar to what players encounter toward the end of a game. Now that your players are in a state of fatigue, you should then organize 20–30 minutes of technical, tactical, and physical drills, exercises that demand powerful actions, quickness, agility, accuracy of passing and shooting and increased tempo from the player.

Evidently, this training plan is specifically designed to improve performance at the end of the game. Such a structure stresses both the physiological aspects of training and the psychological components via maximum nervous system concentration, resilience, willpower, and strong determination.

Model Training for Tactical Pressing

Tactical pressing is not a novelty. On the contrary, it has been used as a tactical weapon for many decades, with two variants being the most popular: 1. total pressing throughout the game, the most taxing physically, and partial pressing during specific parts of the game, often toward the end of the game. Since partial pressing is physiologically the easiest, less taxing variant, it is also considered to be the most effective tactical method. Since total pressing requires an extremely complete and strong conditioning, partial pressing, particularly in the last 10–20 minutes of the game, is recommended using a relatively simple model:

- normal training throughout the session with a visible increase in the
- tempo of every type of training for the last part of the session.

Partial pressing for the last part of the game is suggested in the case of the following game situations:

1. A tie game: high pressing against the opposition with the scope of creating chances to score and win the game.
2. Your team is in the lead, is behind, or must attempt to score the necessary goals to tie or win the game.

Model Training for Controlled Arousal

Coaches are always ready to do the utmost to be successful. No surprise there! To achieve the game objective, to play effectively during games, players must be in a physiological and psychological state of optimal arousal. This physiological and phycological condition of arousal is meant to overcome feelings of excitability and restlessness and reduce anxiety. It can be created by organizing a short workout during the morning (30 minutes). During the pre-game morning practice, coaches have to promote calmness and controlled confidence among their players. Please consider the following model to foster an optimal level of pre-game arousal:

1. Short and light warm-up: 10 minutes.
2. Short, dynamic, fast technical and tactical drills with the ball, and with longer rest intervals than normal: 15 minutes. To avoid the accumulation of fatigue, players can repeat a few powerful, explosive, fast actions, such as few light-weight medicine ball throws, or 2–4 repetitions of reactive jumps, but with a longer rest interval.
3. Cool-down: 5-10 minutes.

Modeling the Microcycle

Model training can also be applied to planning, such as the planning of a microcycle, and weekly training plans with one to two games per week. The first model refers to six microcycles for the early part of the preparatory phase, followed by examples for cycles with one or two games per week.

Note: For each of the following plans we have also proposed how to alternate the energy systems for maximum utilization of your players' energy stores.

Model Training Program for a Six Microcycle Preparatory Phase

Traditionally, the scope of the preparatory phase is to ready the players for all aspects of the game, particularly to build a solid physical foundation with and without the ball, for the league games to follow. Please note that each model of a microcycle specifies days of the week, number of training sessions per day, and the dominant energy system per workout for both the AM and PM sessions.

Aerobic training often follows a free day or very challenging workouts, such as lactic acid/glycolytic energy systems for the purpose of offering players more time to recover and remove fatigue from the system. As exemplified in the following, some training sessions may combine two energy systems, such as alactic/phosphagen, lactic acid/glycolytic with aerobic. Once again, the scope is to alternate energy systems and the intensities used in a given training session, and, as a result, to facilitate compensation and the removal of lactic acid from the system.

You may note that the structure of the week is mentioned in the top of some, such as 3+1 or 5+1. This actually means that for some days of a microcycle there were two planned training sessions: AM and PM. Furthermore, you may plan an even more challenging week, such as 5+1, which means five workouts followed by a half day of free, recovery time. These proposals for two training sessions per day, or five half days of training before a free day are not very popular in soccer. But this type of training is used effectively in many other sports, such as swimming, rowing, and track events. After all, the scope of the preparatory phase is to build a solid fitness capacity, a strong game-specific endurance that will last for the longer part of the league games. One training session per day is not going to improve soccer-specific endurance levels.

Please remember that this type of training is proposed only for the preparatory phase when the scope of training is to achieve strong physical fitness and the improvement of game- and position-specific physical abilities such as strength, power, speed, agility, and endurance. However, some of the proposed microcycles may be altered as per your specific conditions and games schedule.

Table 10.1 Microcycle 1

Day	Mo	Tue	Wed	Th	Fri	Sat	Sun
# of training sessions	1	1	1	1	1	1	0
Energy system	Aerobic	Alactic / Aerobic	Alactic/ Aerobic	Alactic	Aerobic	Lactic acid/ Aerobic	/

Table 10.2 Microcycle 2: 3+1

Day	Mo	Tue	Wed	Th	Fri	Sat	Sun
# of training sessions	2	1	2	1	2	1	0
AM	Alactic	Aerobic	Alactic/ Aerobic	Aerobic	Alactic/ Aerobic	Aerobic	/
PM	Lactic	/	Lactic acid	/	Lactic acid	/	/

Table 10.3 Microcycles 3 and 4: 5+1

Day	Mo	Tue	Wed	Th	Fri	Sat	Sun
# of training sessions	2	2	1	2	2	1	0
AM	Aerobic	Aerobic	Aerobic	Aerobic	Lactic acid/ Aerobic	Aerobic	/
PM	Lactic acid/ Aerobic	Alactic/ Aerobic	/	Lactic acid/ Aerobic	Lactic acid/ Aerobic	/	/

Table 10.4 Microcycles 5 and 6: 3+1

Day	Mo	Tue	Wed	Th	Fri	Sat	Sun
# of training sessions	1	2	1	1	2	1	0
AM	/Physio	Lactic acid/ Tactics/ Aerobic light	/	/Physio	Lactic acid/ Aerobic light	/	/
PM	Aerobic light	Alactic/ Aerobic/ Tactics	Exhibition Game	Aerobic light	Alactic/ Aerobic	Exhibition Game	/

A short note regarding the role of exhibition games

This proposed model does not include exhibition games; instead, it should be planned only when the team is ready, normally toward the end of the preparatory phase. The main scope of exhibition games should not be victory, but rather to test and monitor the readiness of the team, including the effectiveness of each individual player.

Your plan for the exhibition games should be a very progressive selection of your opponents, from a lower standard team to teams from your league. Clear objectives should be set for each exhibition game, such as technical, tactical, and physical, each goal being an intrinsic part of your overall plan for your team. Tactical testing should refer to how lines of players cooperate together, how players from different positions cooperate with their teammates, the effectiveness of transition from offense to defense, and vice versa. At the end of each exhibition game, you should draw your conclusions and decide whether specific changes are necessary.

Note: When you lose, do not lose the lesson!

Model Program for a Microcycle With One Game per Week

The microcycle proposed here (table 10.5) can be a standard format for lower league games, where often there is only one game per week. Please adapt this plan to your own conditions. This plan does not include the role of exhibition games, as briefly discussed previously.

Table 10.5 Suggested training model for a microcycle with one game per week

Day	Mon	Tue	Wed	Th	Fri	Sat	Sun
Training objectives	Post-game recovery, physiotherapy, psychological rehabilitation, and rest	T/TA	T/TA S/P/A/ MxS (30 min)	T/TA longer duration drills	T/TA S/A/ MxS (30 min)	TA model training	Game
Energy systems	/	Aerobic	Alactic/ lactic	Aerobic	Alactic/ lactic	Aerobic light	All
Training demand	/	M	H	M	H	M/L	H

T = technical, TA = tactical, S = speed, P = power, A = agility, MxS = maximum strength, L = light training demand, M = medium training demand, H = high training demand. The time noted for some training (e.g., 30 minutes) refers only to physical aspects of the game.

Model Program for a Microcycle With Two League Games

The structure of the training model for two league games per week is relatively standard when a team has to play two games per week. Prior to and after the game, you have to plan low training demands to rest for the game and facilitate supercompensation.

A major objective of each coach is to remove the fatigue from players' systems via recovery, regeneration, and physiotherapy techniques after a game. A short aerobic activity to produce perspiration may aid in your intent of removing the fatigue from the system since perspiration facilitates the removal of metabolites. As per table 10.6, during league games, the only time you can train maximum speed, agility, power, and maximum strength is at the end of days 2 and 5. This is a maintenance program to keep up the abilities you have trained during the preparatory phase.

Table 10.6 Training model for a microcycle with two games

Day	1	2	3	4	5	6	7
Training objectives	Recovery, regeneration, physiological, psychological	T/TA A/P/ MxS (20 min)	Game	AM: R/R PM: T/TA	T/TA S/P /MxS (20 min)	TA model training	Game
Energy system	/	Alactic/ lactic	All	Aerobic light	Alactic/ lactic	Aerobic light	All
Training demand	/	L/M	H	L	H	L	H

T = technical, TA = tactical, A = agility, P = power, MxS = maximum strength, AM = morning session, RR = recovery, regeneration, psychological rehabilitation, PM = afternoon session, M = medium, H = high, L = low

Modeling a Major Tournament Lasting Two to Three Weeks

Soccer is among many other team sports where championship tournaments, continental, world championships, or the Olympic Games last two to three weeks. During such major championships, some teams play every third day, a schedule that represents a major concern for coaches. These conditions do not refer only to how to prepare for the tournament, but also how to organize daily training and daily activities during an extended game schedule. Table 10.7 illustrates the type of training that may be considered during a major two-week, or longer, tournament.

Table 10.7 Suggested activity during a long tournament

Day	1	2	3	4	5	6	7	8	9	10	11	12
Activity	MT	MT	G	RR O2	MT	G	RR O2	MT	G	RR O2	MT	G

MT = model training: for 45–60 minutes, warm up and rehearse elements of the tactical plan you will use for the next game, G = Game, RR = recovery/regeneration, plus 30 minutes of low-intensity aerobic activity, and simple, low-intensity T and TA training.

Note: Simple low-intensity aerobic training enhances recovery and glycogen restoration much better than an off day with no physical activity at all.

Training Model for the Maintenance of MxS During League Games

Remember the adage what is not trained is detrained! In other words, the MxS you have trained during the preparatory phase has to be maintained during the league games, otherwise everything has been wasted.

Maintenance of MxS is much easier than developing it in the first place. An example of MxS maintenance is presented in tables 10.8 and 10.9.

Table 10.8 Game and MxS schedule in a week with two games

1	2	3	4	5	6	7	8
G		MxS	G		MxS		G

G = game, MxS = maintenance of MxS

Table 10.9 Training program for MxS during the maintenance phase.

Exercise	Load (%)	Number of reps	Number of sets	Rest interval
Calf press	85	3–4	2–3	3
Bench press	80	4	1–2	2–3
Leg press	80	4	2	3

Note: The number of sets suggested for the maintenance (2 sets) and the MxS phase (4 or higher) and for the maintenance program:

- Speed and agility drills are done with the ball.
- Bench press has been selected for maintaining strength of the elbow extension, which is so important for blocking the actions of your opponents in the penalty area.

Conclusions

For any coach, modeling is part of being well organized and a good planner. Preventing unpredictable events or preparing for their negative effects can be beneficial for a soccer coach. This is why we invite you to analyze the above proposals and select what is best for you and the team.

Planning, on the other hand, is an essential tool in soccer training, helping the coach to be well organized and effective in all aspects of the game. As you become more comfortable using these tools, your training will increase its efficiency. In addition, you will also find your own way to express your planning and modeling skills.

CHAPTER 11
DEVELOPING YOUNG SOCCER PLAYERS:
A LONG-TERM APPROACH

The strategy for long-term development of young soccer players must represent one of the major objectives of every national federation and traditional soccer club. There is no future without a strategy of long-term development of young players: from childhood, under 12 (U12) to U23 and national league.

Experienced coaches, technicians with a respected status in the game of soccer, will always agree that players who were exposed to well-organized, systematic training during and after childhood have managed to achieve high and consistent levels of performance. On the other hand, soccer technicians who considered soccer training for children just an imitation of top leagues' programs, who pushed too far and too soon to find new idols, have failed to accomplish their professional dream. We should all remember that young, promising, talented players need time to acquire good soccer-specific skills and physical attributes, such as high levels of speed, agility, power, and resilience.

This is why we invite soccer and S&C coaches to keep in mind that every child evolves at a different rate, and that a child is not a small adult! Children's growth rates, the development of bones, muscles, organs, and nervous systems, are different at different ages, changes from stage to stage, and anatomical, physiological, and psychological evolution substantially dictate a child's performance capabilities.

This is why your training program must consider individual differences and training capabilities. For example, a 14-year-old youth may physically be at the level of a 16-year-old (early developers), whereas another 14-year-old has only the physical capabilities of a 12-year-old player (late developers). Training programs, therefore, need to be individualized according to children's physical (anatomical and physiological) and psychological potential.

Periodization of Long-Term Training

High efficiency in soccer for young players must be based on a well-organized training structure and periodization of long-term training.

To achieve such essential objectives, every national soccer federation along with individual coaches from soccer clubs are invited to create their own periodization of long-term training for their young players. This structure must use the internationally recognized stages of development for U12 to U23 players and must employ advanced training methodology, where technical, tactical, and strength and conditioning training can follow a long-term progression.

Long-term periodization of training is a gradual, progressive physical training development program that, normally, should lead to greater fitness potential without the risk of injury.

Table 11.1 summarizes the concept of long-term periodization in soccer, its two main training objectives, and the scope and type of training for the internationally recognized five stages of development.

Long-Term Training Objectives for Soccer

Long-term training for young players can be divided into two main objectives:

Training Objective 1: Make a child a player (U12–U17)

The main scope of objective 1 is to transform average children into soccer players by exposing them to progressive, well-organized training, where they can acquire and improve fundamental technical skills, the basic elements of tactical training, and the foundational skills of fitness training. Progressive acquisition of basic technical elements of the game can also be divided into technical skills, tactical fundamentals, and physical development.

Technical skills:

- **Learn:** acquire basic skills (U12–U15)
- **Improve** essential skills of soccer (U15–U17)

Tactical fundamentals:

- Understand how the game is played

- Players' positions and their roles on the team
- Basic team strategy: 4-2-4; 4-3-3

Physical development:

- **Learn** to train the basic skills of running, jumping, simple agility, and throwing. Overall physical adaptation to aerobic endurance, basic flexibility, sprinting skill (U12-U15), and the injury-prevention strategy
- **Develop** sprinting speed and agility (U15)
- **Improve** basic strength, power, sprinting speed, speed-endurance (U17)

Training Objective 2: Make a player an athlete (U19 -throughout entire soccer career)

Now that the technical and tactical fundamentals are established, the objective of physical training is to reach the highest athleticism possible. While technical and tactical training have the scope of achieving perfection, physical training will determine whether a player can become the best athlete possible (fast, powerful, agile, and resilient throughout the game).

Technical skills:

- **Continue to improve** essential skills (U19 and throughout players' careers)
- **Improve soccer-specific fitness skills**
- **Perfect** the essential skills of soccer

Tactical training:

- **Variations of team strategies**
- **Offensive strategies:** 4-1-4-1; 3-3-4; etc.
- **Defensive strategies:** 5-3-2, 4-4-2; etc.

Physical training:

- **Develop and improve** MxS, power, abrupt agility, speed endurance
- **Maximize** sprinting speed and agility training under the regimen of energy systems training
- **Maximize** glycolytic and aerobic endurance to improve the rhythm of the game and resilience

Table 11.1 Five stages of long-term development of young players: U12–U23

Main objectives	Stages of development	Scope of training	Type of training
Make a child a player	U 12	Initiation stage	Multilateral
	U 15	Athletic formation stage. Build the foundation of soccer-specific training	Combine multilateral with specific
	U17	Soccer- and position-specific specialized training	Soccer-specific physical training
Make a player an athlete	U19	Transition to high performance	Soccer- and position-specific high athleticism
	U21–23 and over	High performance stage	Position-specific athleticism

As already above, *periodization* originates from the term *period*, which refers to dividing your training into stages, or phases. In the case of youth sports, it refers to five specific phases (stages) of development of soccer-specific physical abilities such as aerobic endurance, flexibility, strength, speed, agility, and game-specific endurance.

The suggested five stages of long-term development (see table 11.1 and the sections that follow) are interconnected in a holistic concept that considers player potential for each age group and assures continuity, progression, and effectiveness.).

U12: Initiation Stage, Selected Methodical Suggestions

Initiation is one of the most important stages in children's involvement in soccer; its success directly depends on the coach's teaching skills and personality. A good coach will have a positive influence on children's decisions to stay in this environment. A negative influence, on the other hand, will increase the number of children who quit the sport. Initiation stage is also called **rapid gains** since children at this age often improve their skills relatively fast.

The following suggestions should assist you in generating training programs important for the development of soccer-specific abilities: technical skills, overall fitness development, and resilience.

The proposed suggestions refer to three essential elements in soccer: 1) technical, 2) physical (fitness), and 3) psychological and social. These elements are taught in a logical progression:

1. **learning**, or the acquisition of technical skills during the early part of children's involvement in soccer
2. **improving** the rate fundamental soccer skills advance
3. **perfecting**, the ultimate stage which highlights soccer skills desired by every player

1 Technical

- Offer children the necessary time and conditions to individually work on basic soccer skills (ball control, accuracy of passing/shooting, target passing, etc.).
- Design drills and number of repetitions that children can perform with ease. Encourage children to focus on repeating each drill correctly, with best technique possible.
- Promote experimental learning by giving children opportunities to design their own drills, games, and other activities. Encourage them to use their imaginations and be creative.
- Simplify or modify the size of the field and rules to help children understand and enjoy the game.
- During the game, consider introducing young players to situations that demonstrate the importance of teamwork.
- Teach the players not only all the techniques and tactics of the game but also the specific position they play in the team. House leagues are an ideal environment for younger age groups to learn these skills because they can practice in a low-stress environment.
- Involve children in multi-skills training that can improve coordination and technical acquisition which is so essential for technical improvement.

2 Fitness

- During the early part of training, children must be exposed to a progressive, low-intensity training program that fits their training potential.
- Exercises should follow a simple progression from simple to complex, from a training program easy to tolerate to one that increases progressively in difficulty.
- Encourage the development of an overall cardiorespiratory fitness training that progressively helps a child to more easily tolerate fatigue.
- Strength training must begin with simple, low-intensity and low-load exercises to ensure a progressive adaptation of ligaments, tendons, and muscles to build a progressive foundation for developing strength, power, speed ,and agility. Without this base, injuries may show up far too early in a player's career.
- Strength training with lower loads should ensure a multilateral, overall physical development of the body.
- Multilateral, multi-skills training enriches skill experience. As a result, it dramatically improves coordination, which is so essential for skill development.
- Young players should also practice other sports recreationally, specifically swimming, since this sport is also an environment that develops the cardiorespiratory system while minimizing the stress on joints, ligaments, and connective tissues.
- Injury-prevention strategy: Coaches should also consider that during early stages bones are still fragile. Ends of bones are still cartilaginous and in the process of calcifying. Therefore, bones might be susceptible to injuries.

3 Psychological and Social

- Children at this stage have a low attention span, may experience difficulty concentrating on a task, and fatigue quickly. Yet they are action oriented. Consequently, keep theoretical explanation to a minimum.
- Ensure fun, enjoyment, and socializing with teammates. This is very important for most of the children involved in soccer.
- Praise children who are punctual, orderly, and have self-discipline.
- Use variety and creativity to stimulate their attention and concentration.

- Create the environment for boys and girls to participate together on the same team.
- Ensure children enjoy your training.
- Encourage children to participate in different games.
- Encourage participation in other sports as well to socialize with other children.
- Design drills, games, and activities to maximize children's opportunities for active participation.

U15: Player Formation Stage

The U15 stage represents a transition from a low intensity (U12) to another stage (U17), where the intensity and training demand can be slightly increased. This transition is called the *player formation stage*, since it readies the players for a more complex, soccer- and position-specific technical, tactical, and physical training.

At this stage, however, most players are still vulnerable to injuries, particularly if coaches believe in the adage of *no pain, no gain*. Whole physical development, particularly the cardiorespiratory system, has to be continuously increased, so that players can easier tolerate the build-up of lactic acid in the system, specifically during higher-intensity games.

During U15, young players experience variations in individual differences in growth and development, so players' performances can visibly vary for few more years. Please also consider that some players may experience rapid growth spurts of up to 5 inches (12 cm), which can cause disturbances in coordination and strength potential (legs grow and change the proportions between body parts). If you experience these instances, calmness and patience can be important attributes for both players and coaches. Coaches' patience is even more necessary when precision, coordination, and accuracy of skills are more important than winning.

Accurate passing, shooting, and the timing of most technical executions continue to improve during U15. Attention should be paid to the differences between early- and late-maturing young players. Those who mature early may experience temporary lapses in motor coordination, which may temporarily affect skill accuracy and good coordination of some physical actions (Sharma and Hirtz, 1991; Skinner and Piek, 2001; Caprinica and Millard-Stafford, 2011; Bompa and Carrera, 2015).

To overcome such challenges, you should expose those who mature early to additional time and variety of exercises to improve coordination, rhythm, and spatial orientation. In time, improvements will occur, and players will learn how to control their actions and skills.

The following guidelines are listed in a specific progression, without specifying the field, as we did for U12 program. However, our suggestions will help you design your own training programs appropriate for the athletic formation stage:

- Expose your players to soccer-specific drills, simple tactical maneuvers that will assist them in increasing both the volume and intensity of training.
- To maximize specificity, repeat most drills with the ball.
- Introduce drills that will help players reinforce skill development and the essential tactics of the game.
- Create a well-developed aerobic base that will help your players to effectively cope with the build-up of lactic acid and its negative effects, both physical and psychological, particularly toward the end of both halves of the game.
- Create specific and diverse drills with the aim of improving range of motion and specifically to develop flexibility of ankle, knee, and hip joints.
- Create drills that develop coordination, attention control, and reaction and movement time.
- Use challenging technical and tactical drills that increase fatigue and reproduce physiological and psychological conditions similar to the end of a game.
- Progressively introduce more demanding exercises that develop general strength, power, sprinting speed, agility, cardiorespiratory endurance, and game resilience.
- Remember to emphasize fun! Children enjoy having fun during training. Use your imagination to create variety, particularly when players experience fatigue.
- Always remember to set aside the necessary time for socializing with teammates. That makes your players happy, and they will enjoy training more.

U17: Specialization Stage

The specialization stage represents the time when players are exposed to the more specific elements of training, the higher technical, tactical, physical, and psychological training demands, and must increase their ability to better tolerate stress and fatigue. All aspects of training for this stage must be game and position specific and specialized. Similarly, special attention must also be paid to the intensity and the volume of training. Please always remember that compared to many other types of soccer training, high-intensity training is a higher injury risk for players.

U17 is also the stage when players have already acquired all the technical fundamentals of the game. From now on, coaches' objectives must be technical finesse, perfecting all the game- and position-specific techniques, and ensuring that players are able to play effectively with both legs.

The role of the coach also changes during the specialization stage from a teaching to a primarily training role.

As children approach developmental stages post puberty and adolescence, certain abilities have a different rate of development. Coordination that had slower improvement during puberty will now continue to improve at a constant rate.

The following guidelines will help you design training programs that are suitable for your players at the specialization stage:

- While U17 is clearly a soccer-specialization stage, the coach can still expose his or her players to varied, multi-skill drills that can increase sprinting speed, agility, strength, power, and game- and position-specific endurance.
- Keep focusing on the technical and tactical refinement of the game and position. Now is the time to stress specificity.
- Closely monitor how players are coping with increased physical and psychological demands. They can be vulnerable to overtraining!
- While training and game demand increase so too will players' self-awareness. Some of the more talented players may develop a superiority complex, whereas the others who struggle to keep up with training and game demands may isolate themselves and lose confidence. This is why

coaches must create a friendly environment, team cohesion, and confidence in every player. Players must know that the coach believes every player has unique qualities and potential. And that every player's first goal is The Team.

- One should not be surprised that those players who struggle today might become the stars of tomorrow's team.
- Soccer and S&C coaches must constantly monitor players' rates of improvement in the known soccer-dominant abilities: power, sprinting speed, agility, dynamic flexibility, and game-, and position-specific endurance.
- Repeat specific tactical drills with higher intensity and rhythm similar to a game.
- Higher intensity and rhythm of the game always results in fatigue. While this is a natural outcome you should try to avoid exhaustion. So constantly monitor players' reactions to your training and use recovery and regeneration techniques to remove fatigue before the next training session or game.
- As much as possible involve players in your decision-making process.
- Although you may still continue the use of nonspecific training, particularly during the preparatory phase, most training activities (physical and technical or tactical) should be game and position specific.
- Offer your players the opportunity to learn the theoretical aspects of training and the game.
- Make sure that S&C coaches use specific strength training where the selected exercises address the prime movers that perform the dominant soccer actions: running, sprinting, agility, and jumping. Avoid strength-training programs that use fewer than four repetitions, since players at this stage are not ready to use heavy loads (or loads over 80% of 1RM).
- Expose your players to simple, stress-free, easy-to-perform plyometric exercises with a duration of 4–12 seconds (skipping rope, jumping over low benches or hurdles) and a longer rest interval (2 min).
- Plan tactical drills where both the anaerobic and glycolytic energy system are used. From this point on, players are capable of tolerating the build-up of lactic acid.
- Make sure that technical drills are biomechanically correct and physiologically efficient.
- Try to constantly use individual and team tactics. Make sure they are interesting and challenging.

- Stimulate technical variety, prolong concentration, anticipation, initiative, self-control, quick decision-making processes, competitive vigor, and fair play.
- Organize shooting practice with maximum concentration and improved precision.
- Remind your players that although important **winning isn't everything**.

U19: Transition to the High-Performance Stage

U19 represents an important stage as players mature to progressively achieve technical and tactical skill perfection. These essential goals are possible by reducing the time U17 has devoted to overall technical/tactical and physical training and instead use the time to perfect technical skills that are necessary in order to achieve high performance.

From this stage on, the scope of training is to concentrate on improving and perfecting all technical/tactical elements of soccer, and as well as technical and tactical effectiveness. By the end of this stage, most players have finished growing, and many aspects of physical training are more accessible.

Before attempting to create a good training program for U19 players, consider the following suggestions:

- Start emphasizing technical and tactical training as per the physiological specificity of the game and position played.
- Increase players' ability to tolerate higher training demand by designing a training program that taxes all energy systems present in soccer.
- Organize your training based on the concept of energy systems training. For maximum physiological compensation, you have to alternate training sessions emphasizing different energy systems. Example: a training session emphasizing the glycolytic energy system must be followed by a session where a lower demand of aerobic endurance is trained.
- Introduce specific training to continue to improve strength, power, agility, sprinting speed, and game- and position-specific endurance.
- Introduce technical and tactical training as per the concept of energy system training.

- Attempt to increase the intensity of training to higher levels than used during U17.
- Use the same approach regarding training volume, duration, and distance covered in training. Increase training demand as it refers to the rhythm of the game.
- Combine tactical drills with psychological objectives: good timing, tenacity, maximum concentration, quick reaction during all aspects of the game, and a high willingness and determination to win.
- Practice and emphasize fast transitions from defense to offense and offense to defense.
- Plan periodic testing once a month, especially during the preparatory phase, as well as formal tests to monitor physical improvement to your training: maximum speed, agility, MxS, power, and specific endurance.
- Always ensure your players are ready for your training session. Explain training objectives and ask for your players' opinions.
- Plan maximum sprinting speed with and without the ball.
- Have a special session with your players regarding good sports nutrition and meal plans. You may also invite a nutritionist.
- Ensure that the S&C coach emphasizes the development of MxS 60 to 80% of 1RM. Please remember that power, agility, and sprinting speed directly depend on your players' levels of MxS. Also introduce bounding exercises (triple jump drills like those used in track and field), which are very effective for game-specific power actions.
- The first post-game training session must emphasize recovery, regeneration, rehabilitation, and, if necessary, physiotherapy treatment.

U21 to U23: High-Performance Stage

U21-23 is the time when players can maximize their performance and convert the pillars of soccer—technical and tactical perfection, physical improvement, and psychological fortitude—into the highest physiological efficiency.

Coaches should aim to increase players' technical refinement to effectively use technical improvements during the tactical complexity of drills and games. Employ tactical drills to also improve specific speed and endurance, both anaerobic (phosphagen and glycolytic) and aerobic (oxidative).

These two classifications of player development (U21-U23) represent the entrance of most players into the world of high performance, high professionalism, and the apex of athletic satisfaction. The main differences between the two classifications exist in intensity or load of power and strength training, and the individual ability to tolerate work. As you begin to create specific training programs for top players, please consider the following guidelines:

- Refine and improve game-specific and position-specific technical finesse in all aspects of the sport or game.
- Use an energy systems stratagem to maximize game- and position specific training.
- Based on the previous, create a fitness training program that aligns with your players' capabilities and the level achieved by the players from your league: MxS, power, sprinting speed, speed endurance, agility, and specific aerobic system.
- Design game- and position-specific tactical drills based on the proportions of energy systems dominant in soccer. These drills should result not only in the improvement of your team's tactical efficiency but must also be adapted to the duration of each system:

1. Phosphagen: High intensity, maximum speed, and agility with and without the ball for a duration of 8–12 seconds.
2. Glycolytic: A duration of 30–45 seconds but using high intensity.
3. Oxidative: Medium-intensity aerobic-dominant tactical drills using several players and mimicking transitions from defense to offense and from offense to defense (1-3/5 minutes).

- Use tactical drills for the specific purpose of developing lactic acid tolerance to overcome fatigue (30-45 or longer seconds). These drills should be tactically complex and use several players to also improve players' psychological capacity and will power.
- Create technical and tactical drills in which players are exposed to improving the quality of the game, rhythm of play, pacing and timing, and react to your opponents' offensive and defensive tactics.
- Try to constantly monitor player improvement and reaction to your training programs.

- Focus your training on what is important in soccer, not on the latest training gadgets or what is currently popular.

Selected Long-Term Models for the Periodization of Strength, Speed, Agility, and Endurance

Throughout the long-term development of young players, specific guidelines for the periodization of strength, speed, agility, and endurance can be used (tables 11.2–11.5). Please use your own expertise to practically apply these suggested guidelines throughout the traditional stages of development to ensure the necessary physical development of your players, from U12 to U21–23, and over.

Table 11.2 Periodization of strength training from U12–U23

Stage of development	U12	U15	U17	U19	U21–23
Scope of strength training	Initiation in the fundamentals of strength training, injury prevention using exercises that address most muscle groups	A Injury prevention Simple Ag P	A P Ag	A MxS (low loads) P PE Ag	A MxS P Ag ME

A = adaptation, P = power, Ag = agility, MxS = maximum strength, PE = power endurance, ME = muscular endurance

Table 11.3 Periodization of speed for U12 to U23

Stage of development	U12	U15	U17	U19	U21–23
Energy system	Aerobic Alactic	All three energy systems	All three	All three	All three
Types of training	Learning specific and nonspecific running skills	All forms of acceleration Alactic maximum speed	All forms of maximum acceleration and deceleration	All forms of maximum acceleration and deceleration with high intensity	All forms of maximum acceleration and deceleration with high intensity

Table 11.4 Periodization of agility training

Stage of development	U12	U15	U17	U19	U21	U23
Type of strength	A	A P	A, P MxS (50-60%)	MxS (60-70%) P	MxS (60-80%) P PE	MxS (70-90%) P PE
Ag Energy systems	Ag: Learn simple drills, alactic	Ag: Increase difficulty, alactic, introduce lactic drills	Ag: Difficult drills, alactic Difficult Alactic Low–medium intensity, aerobic drills	Ag: Difficult drills, all three energy systems	Ag: All energy systems Medium–high intensity	Ag: Complex drills, all energy systems

Table 11.5 Periodization of endurance training

Stage of	U12	U15	U17	U19	U 21-23
Scope of training	Drills for aerobic	Drills for aerobic, alactic	Game- and position-specific drills for all three energy systems	Same type of specific training	Same type of specific training

CONCLUSION

Please analyze some of the suggested training programs and adapt these suggestions in your training. However, more importantly, create your own programs as per the specifics of your players and league games.

For those involved in training younger players (U12–U15) please assess all factors that can affect your training: growth and development, social, psychological, medical, and nutrition.

Enjoy what your profession is offering you. It is a great profession. However, equally important is to be proud of what you are offering to others, particularly to the young players: your talent and love for soccer.

Please accept our deepest respect for your work and professionalism.

GLOSSARY

acceleration: The ability to increase movement action or velocity in a minimal amount of time.

actin: A protein involved in muscle contraction.

adaptation: Positive changes in the functions of the body as a result of training.

adenosine triphosphate (ATP): A complex chemical compound formed with the energy released from food and stored in muscle cells.

aerobic energy system: The primary source of ATP during low-intensity, long-duration physical activity.

agility: The ability of a player to quickly change direction during the game. It is a highly desirable quality in most team sports, particularly in offence and for playmakers. Agility is clearly enhanced by and strongly dependent on a player's level of strength and maximum strength.

alactic (phosphagen) energy system: An anaerobic (i.e., without the presence of oxygen) energy system that provides energy for short-term (less than 12 seconds) activity.

alactic energy system: The energy system that provides energy via the breakdown of glucose without the presence of oxygen. It supplies energy for 20 seconds to 2 minutes.

anaerobic: In the absence of oxygen.

biological age: An indication of age based upon sexual maturation.

biomotor and motor abilities: The physical abilities used in a sport (agility, flexibility, speed, strength, and endurance).

carbohydrate: A basic foodstuff; a compound composed of carbon, hydrogen, and oxygen.

chronological age: The actual age of an individual.

concentric contraction: The shortening of a muscle during contraction.

cross bridges: Extensions of myosin.

density: The number of training activities performed per unit of time.

detraining: A reversal of adaptation to exercise caused by a longer duration of inactivity.

eccentric contraction: The lengthening of a muscle during contraction.

discharge rate: The magnitude of neural activation and the subsequent force displayed by a muscle.

endurance: The capacity to perform work for an extended period of time.

energy: The capacity to perform work.

energy system: One of the three metabolic systems involving a series of chemical reactions which form waste products and manufacture ATP.

ergogenesis: The proportion, expressed in percentage, of the three energy systems that supply energy for a given sport.

extension: Stretching a joint.

fast-twitch fibers (FT): A muscle fiber characterized by fast contraction time beneficial to speed, power, and agility activities.

fatigue: A state of discomfort and decreased efficiency resulting from training.

flexibility: The range of motion about a joint.

flexion: Bending a joint.

glycogen: A storage form of carbohydrate that is found in the skeletal muscle and liver.

glycolytic (lactic acid) energy system: The end product of the fast glycolytic system; replenishes ATP without the presence of oxygen; and is associated with high level of fatigue.

hypertrophy: An increase in the size of the muscles as a result of a strength-training program.

innervation number: The number of muscle fibers innervated (activated) by a single motor unit.

intensity of training: The qualitative element of training such as speed, agility, power, and maximum strength.

intermittent work: Exercise performed with alternating periods of relief and rest.

interval training: A physical activity interrupted by a rest interval; mostly used during training of the anaerobic and aerobic systems.

isometric (static) contraction: Muscle contraction in which tension develops with no changes in length.

isotonic contraction: Muscle contraction in which it is shortening and lengthening; also known as dynamic contractions.

jumping power: The capacity of the leg extensors muscles to apply force against the ground and jump as high as possible. The higher the leg power, the higher the jump capacity of an athlete.

lactate: A salt formed from lactic acid that has to be eliminated from the system before an athlete can return to maximum efficiency.

lactic acid (glycolytic): See glycolytic energy system.

macrocycle: A training plan 4–6 weeks in duration.

maturation: Progress towards adulthood.

maximum strength: The highest force an athlete can lift or overcome during one maximal contraction. Often it is also called one-repetition maximum, or 1RM.

metabolism: The sum of the (anabolic and catabolic) reactions occurring in the body.

metabolite: Any substance produced by a metabolic reaction.

microcycle: A training plan for one week.

minute volume: The volume of air inhaled and exhaled into and from the lungs per minute.

motor unit: The motor nerve and the muscle fibers it innervates.

movement time: The capacity of an athlete to quickly move a limb.

myosin: A protein involved in muscular contraction.

myotatic stretch reflex: A muscle contraction in response to the stretching within a muscle.

one-repetition maximum (1RM): See maximum strength.

overtraining: A decrement of performance caused by overwork.

oxidative (aerobic) energy system: See aerobic energy system.

oxygen system: The primary source of ATP at rest and during long, low-intensity exercise. It requires oxygen to produce energy and is also known as the aerobic system.

oxygen debt or oxygen deficit: The anaerobic contribution to the total energy cost of an activity.

periodization: A systematic sequencing of training phases during a training plan. The same concept is also valid for planning the development of physical abilities, such as strength, speed, agility, and endurance.

power: Unit of work expressed per unit of time (power = work/time); often considered a factor of intensity. It refers to work where speed and strength are the main contributors.

power endurance: The capacity to apply a nonstop power action for a longer time.

physiology: A branch of biology; the study of living organs and the whole human body during physical activity.

phosphagen: A group of compounds, collectively refers to ATP and CP (creatine phosphate).

phosphagen energy system: See alactic energy system.

plyometrics: Drills using an explosive–reactive type of exercise. Often called jump training.

prime movers: Main muscles performing the main technical skills.

proprioceptors: Monitor the position and status of the neuromuscular system.

reaction time: The time it takes the neuromuscular system to respond to a stimulus (athletic action).

recovery (exercise recovery): A pause between bouts of training that replenishes energy.

rest interval: The pause, in minutes or seconds, taken during speed, agility, strength, and endurance training.

set: The total number of repetitions an athlete performs before taking a rest interval or pause.

slow-twitch fibers (ST): Muscle fibers characterized by slow contraction time, low anaerobic capacity, and high aerobic capacity, making it suited to low power output activities.

speed: The ability to cover a given distance in the shortest period of time (run, swim, etc.).

speed endurance: The ability to maintain a high level of speed for a longer period. For instance, in a 100 m race, the ability to maintain high velocity in the last 20 m depends on the level of speed endurance. In team sports, speed endurance also refers to the ability to repeat many sprints at high velocity.

strength: The force generated by muscle contractions.

stretching–shortening cycle: A combination of eccentric and concentric muscle actions.

super compensation: Also known as the general adaptation syndrome, it refers to the body's response to stressors and how it adapts to them.

training: An exercise program to develop an athlete for a game.

training demand: A summation of all the factors used in training and games.

volume of training: High amount of work in all aspects of training and the game.

REFERENCES

Ade J., J. Fitzpatrick, and P.S. Bradley. 2016. AE. High-intensity efforts in elite soccer matches and associated movements patterns, technical skills and tactical actions. Information for position-specific training drills. 2016. *J Sports Sci* 34:2205-2214.

Aquino R., L.H.P Vieira, C. Carling et al. 2017. Effects of competitive standard, team formation and playing position on match running performance of Brazilian professional soccer players. *Int. J Perform Anal Sport.* 17: 695-705.

Aoyagi K., J. He et al. 2018. Nov. A subgroup of chronic low back pain patients with central sensitization. *Clin J Pain* 35 (11): 869-879.

Andrzejewski M., J. Chmura, B. Pluta, S. Ryszard, K. Andrzej. August 2013. Analysis of sporting activities of professional soccer players. *J Str and Condi Res* 27(8): 2134-2140.

Ashton-Miller, J.A., E.M. Wojtys, L.J. Huston, and D. Fry-Welch. 2001. Can proprioception be improved by exercise? *Knee Surgery Sports Traumatology Arthroscopy* 9 (3): 128-36.

Avalos, M., P. Hellad, and J.C. Chatard. May 2003. Modeling the training-performance relationship using mixed model in elite swimmers. *Med Sci Sports Exerc* 35(5):833-46.

Bangsbo, J. 1994. Energy demands in competitive soccer. *J Sports Sci.* 12: 5-12.

Bangsbo, J., F.M. Iaia, and P. Krustrup. 207 Metabolic response and fatigue in soccer. Int J of Sports Physiol and Performance. 2 (2): 111-27.

Bangsbo, J. 2014. Physiological demand of football. *Spots Sci. Exchange.* 27 (125): 1-6.

Benis, R., M. Bonato, A. La La Torre. Sep 2016. Elite female basketball players' body-weight neuromuscular training and performance in the Y-balance test. *J Ath Train* 51 (9): 688-695.

Blazevich, A. Aug 2, 2021. Muscles are important, but stiff tendons are the secret ingredient for high-speed performance. *The Conversation EDT* 1.20.

Bloomfield, J., R. Polman, P. O'Donoghue. 2007. Physical demands of different positions in FA Premier League Soccer *J Sports Sci Med*. Mar 6 (1): 63-70.

Bohm S., F. Hersmann, and A. Arampatzis. 2015. Human tendon adaptation in response to mechanical loading: a systematic review and meta-analysis of exercise intervention studies in healthy adults. *Sports Med-Open*. Doi/10-1186/s40798-015-0009-9.

Bompa, T.O. 1983. *Theory and methodology of training*. Kendal/Hunt Publishing Company.

Bompa, T.O. and C. Francis. 1995. Personal notes on testing Canadian sprinter at Biomechanics Laboratory, York University, Toronto, ON. Canada.

Bompa, T. 2006. *Total training for coaching team sports*. Sport books publisher. Toronto, ON. Canada.

Bompa, T. 2009. *Periodization: Theory and methodology of training*. Champaign, IL. Human Kinetics.

Bompa, T.O. and M. Carrera. 2015. *Conditioning young athletes*. Champaign, IL. Human Kinetics.

Bompa, T.O. and C Buzzichelli. 2019. *Periodization of strength training for sports*. Champaign, IL. Human Kinetics.

Bompa, T.O. and S.O. Sarandan. 2023. *Training and conditioning young athletes*. Champaign, IL. Human Kinetics.

Bradley, P.S., C. Lago-Penas, E. Rey, and A. Gomez Diaz. 2013. The effect of high and low percentage ball possession on physical and technical profiles in English FA Premier League soccer matches. *J Sports Sci* 31 (12): 1261–1270.

Bush M., C. Barnes, D.T. Archer, B. Hogg, and P.S. Bradley. 2015. Evaluation of match performance parameters for various playing positions in the English Premier League. *Hum MovSci* 39: 1–11.

Capranica, L. and M.L. Millard-Stafford. 2011. Youth sport specialization: How to manage competition and training *Int. J. Sports Physiol. Perform.* 6(4): 572–579.

Clark K.P. and P.G. Weyand. Sept 14, 2014. Are running speed maximised with simple sprint stand mechanic? *J Appl Physiol* 117 (6): 604–15.

Churchill, S.M., G. Trewartha, I.N. Bezodis, and A.I.T. Salo. 25 Sept. 2015. Force production during maximal effort bend sprinting: Theory vs. reality. *Scan J of Medicine Sci in Sports*. 26(10): 1171–1179.

Colyer, S.L., R. Nagahara, Y. Takai, and A.I.T. Sato. 2018. How sprinters accelerate beyond the velocity plateau of soccer players: waveform analysis of ground reaction forces. *Scand J Med Sci Sports* 28 (12): 2527–2535.

Cushion, C. 2007 Dec. Modelling the complexity of the coaching process. *IntJ of Sports Sci & Coaching* 2(4) Doi/10.1260/174795407783359650.

Cyrenne, P. and H. Grant. 2009. Economics of decision making. *Economics of education review.* 28(2): 237–248.

Dambroz, F., F.M. Clemente, and I. Teoldo. 2022. The effect of physical fatigue on the performance of soccer players: A systematic review. *Plos One* 17 (7):e0270099.

Dellal, A., K. Chamari, D.P. Wong, S. Ahmadi, D. Keller, R. Barros, G.N. Biscotti, and C. Carling. 2011. Comparison of physical and technical performance in European soccer match-play: FA Premier League and La Liga. *Eur J Spor Sc.* 11 (1): 51–59.

Di Mascio, M., and P.S. Bradley. 2013. Evaluation of the most intense high-intensity running period in English FA premier league soccer matches. *J Strength Cond Res* 27: 909–916.

Di Salvo, V., R. Baron, H. Tscham et al. 2007. Performance characteristics according to playing position in elite soccer. *Int J Sports Med* 28: 222–227.

D'Lima D.D., B.J. Freglyet al. Feb 2012. Knee joint forces: prediction, measurement, and significance. *Pro Inst Med Eng* 226 (2): 95–102.

Dolci A. and M. Pentheghini. May 2014. Harmonization of automated hemolysis index assessment and use: It is possible? *Clinica Chimica Acta.* 32: 38-43.

Dolci F., N.H. Hart, A.E. Kilding, P. Chivers, B. Piggott, and T. Spiteri. June 2020. Physical and energetic demand in soccer: A brief review. *Str and Condi J.* 42 (3): 70–78.

Dorn, T.W., A.G. Schache, M.G. Pandy. 2012. Muscular strategy shift in human running: dependence of running speed on hip and ankle muscle performance. *J Exp Biolog.* 215: 1944–56.

Dorn, J.W., A.G. Schache, M.G. Pandy. Oct 21. 2019. What muscles are moving us while we run? *J of Exp Biology* 215: 1944–1956.

Duchateau J.,S. Severine, B. Stephane., and A. Carpentier. Jan 2021. Strength training: in search of optimal strategies to maximise neuromuscular performance: exercise and sports sciences review. Jan 2021. Doi: 10.1249/JES.0234.

Dupont, G., M.A. Nedelec, A. McCall and N.A. Maffiuletti. 2018. Football recovery strategy. *Aspetar Sports Med Journal.* Volume 4.

Ekstrand, J., M. Hagglund, and M. Walden. 2011. Epidemiology of muscle injuries in professional football. *Am J Sports Med* (June). 39 (6): 1226–32.

Ekstrand, J., A. Spreco, H. Bengtsson, and R. Bahr. 2021. Injury rates decreased in men's professional football: an 18-year prospective cohort study of almost 12,000 injuries sustained during 1.8 million hours of play. *British J of Sports Med* 55, Issue 19.

Ekstrand, J., H. Bengstrom, M. Walden, M. Davison, K.M. Khan, and M. Hagglund. 2023.Hamstring injury rates have increased during recent seasons and now constitute 24% of all injuries in men's professional football: the UEFA elite clubs injury study from 2021–2022. *Br.J. Sports Med.* 57: 292–298.

Elliasen, W., A.H. Saeterbakken, and R. van den Tiilart. Aug 2018. Comparison of bilateral and unilateral squats exercises on barbell kinematics and muscle activation. *Int J of Sports Phys Therapy.* 13 (5): 871–81.

Ekblom, B. 1986 Jan. Fed. Applied physiology of soccer. *Sports Med.* 3(1): 50–60.

Enoka, R.M. 1994. *Neuromechanical basis of kinesiology.* 2nd ed. Champaign, IL: Human Kinetics.

Enoka, R.M. 2015. *Neuromechanics of human movement.* 4th ed. Champaign IL: Human Kinetics.

Escamila, R.F., G.S. Fleisig et al. Sep12 2001. Effects of technique variations on knee biomechanics during the squat and leg press. *Med Sci Sports Exerc.* 33 (9): 1552-66.

Faude, O., T. Koch, and T. Meyer. 2012. Straight sprinting is the most frequent action in goal situations in professional football. *J Sports Sci* 30: 625-631.

Ferris, R.M. and DA Hawkins.13 July 2020. Gastrocnemius and soleus muscles contributions to ankle plantar flexion torque as a function of ankle and knee angle. *Sports injuries & Medicine*: 4:163. Doi: 10.29011/2576-9596.100063.

Fisher, J., J. Steele, et al. Sep. 2011. Evidence-based resistance training recommendations. *Medicina Sportiva.* 15: 147-162.

Fox, E.L. 1984. *Sports Physiology.* New York. CBS College.

Hagglund, M., M. Waldau, and J. Ekstrand.2013. Risk factors for lower extremities muscle injury in professional soccer: The UEFA Injury Study. *Am.J. Sports Med.* 2013:41 (2):327-35.

Hagglund, M. and M. Walden. 2016. Risks factors for acute knee injury in female youth football. Knee Surgery Sports Traumatol Arthrosc. 24 (3):737-46.

Hagglund M. 2023. Rates of injuries in football., Home Page. University of Linkoping. Sweden.

Hamner, S.R., A. Seth, and S.L. Delo. 2010. Muscle contribution o propulsion and support during running. J 43(14): 2709-2716.

Hands, D.E. and X.J. de Jonge. June 2020. Current time-motion analyses of professional football methods in top level domestic leagues: a systematic review. *Int J Perf Analysis in Sports.* 20(5): 7474-765.

Harrison, J.M. and V.F. Rafuse. Nov. 2020. Muscle fiber-type specific terminal Schwann cell pathology leads to sprouting deficits following partial denervation inSOD1mice. *Neurobiology of Disease.* 145. Doi/10.1016/j.nbd.2020.105052.

Herbert, R.D. and M. Gabriel. 2002. Effects of stretching before and after exercising on muscle soreness and risk of injury: A systematic review. *Br. Med. J.* 325: 468-70.

Hernadez-Moreno, J., V. Castro et al. 2011. Game rhythm and stoppages in soccer: A case study from Spain. *J of Human Sports and Exercise* 6 (4). Doi: 10.100/jhse.2011.64.03.

Hughes, M., T. Caudrelier et al. 2012. Moneyball and soccer: an analysis of the key performance indicators in elite male soccer players by position. *J Human Sport and Ex.*7(2): 402–412.

Hughes, D.C., S. Ellefsen, and K. Baar. 2018 Jun. Adaptation to endurance and strength. *CSH Perspective in Medicine* 8 (6): a029769.

Ingraham, S.J. 2003. The role of flexibility in injury prevention and athletic performance: Have we stretched the truth? *Minnesota Med.* 86(5): 58–61.

Kohl, H.W. III and H.D. Cook, eds. 2013. *Educating the student body: Taking physical activity and physical education to school.* Washington, D.C.: National Academic Press.

Khuu, A., E. Foch, and C. Lewis. Apr. 2016. Not all single leg squats are equal: A biomechanical comparison of three variations. I *J of Sports Therapy.* 11 (2): 201–211.

Kunrath, C.A., F. da Silva et al. 2020. Mental fatigue in soccer: a systematic review. *Rev Bras Med Esporto.* 26 (2) doi/10.1590/1517.

Laursen, P.B., and D.G. Jenkins. The scientific basis for high-intensity interval training: optimising training programmes and maximising performance in highly trained endurance athletes. *Sports Med* 32:53-73, 2002.

Law, B., P. Post, and P. McCulllagh. 2017, Dec 19. Modeling in sports performance: Oxford research encyclopedias. Psychology. Doi/10.1093/acrefor. 9780190236557.013,159.

Luc, P., C. Couprie et al. 2009. Semantic segmentation using adversarial networks. Cornell University. ArXive. Doi/10.48550/arXiv 1611.08400.

McCurdy, K., G.A. Langford et al. Sep 1, 2004. The reliability of 1- and3RM tests of unilateral strength in trained and untrained men and women. *J Sports Sci Med.* (3):190-6.

McDonagh, M., and C.T.M. Davies. 1984. Adaptive response of mammalian skeletal muscle to exercise with high loads. *European Journal of Applied Physiology* 52: 139–55.

Mero, A., P.V. Komi, and R.J. Gregor. 1992 June, and 2015 Oct. 14. Biomechanics of sprint running. A review. *Sports Med* 13 (6): 376–92.

Mohr, M., P. Krustrup, and J. Bangsbo. 2003. Match performance of high-performance soccer players with special reference to development of fatigue. *J Sports Sci* 21: 519–528.

Mohr, M., P. Krustrup, and J. Bangsbo. 18 Feb. 2007. *J sports Sci.* 23(6) : 593–599.

Monte, A., V. Baltzopoulos, C.N. Maganaris, and P. Zamparo. 2020. Medialis and vastus lateralis in vivo muscles tendon behaviour during running at increased speed. *Scand J of Medicine & Sci in sports.* 30 (7): 163–76.

Morgan, R. and G. Adamson. 1959. *Circuit training.* London: G. Bell and sons.

Morgan, R., P. Orme, L. Anderson, and B. Drust. 2014. Principles and practice of training for soccer. *Science Direct.* Doi/10.1016/j.jshs.2014.07.002.

Morin, J.B., P. Gimenez, P. Edouard, and A.P. 2015. Arnal: Sprint acceleration mechanics: the major role of hamstrings in horizontal force production. *Frontier in Physiology*, 6 (404).

Neptune, R.R. and K. Sasaki. March 2005. Ankle plantar flexor force production is an important determinant of the preferred walk-to-run transmission speed. *J Exp Biol* 208(5): 799–808.

Pandy, M.G., A.K.M. Lai, A.G. Schache, and Yi-Chung Lin. 16 July 2021. How muscles maximise performance in accelerated sprinting. *Scan J of Medicine & Sci in Sports.* 31 (10): 1882–1896.

Perroni, F., G.P. Emereziani, et al. 2019. Energy cost and energy sources of an elite female soccer player to repeated sprint ability test: A case study. *The Open Sports Science Journal.* 12: 10–16.

Popescu, O. 1958. Refacerea dupa effort (Post-training recovery). Bucuesti. *Stadion:* 23–28.

Powers, S. and E. Howley. 2011. *Exercise Physiology: Theory and application to fitness and performance.* McGraw-Hill.

Rampinini, E., A. Sassi, et al. Jan 2020. Physiological determinants of Yo-Yo intermittent recovery tests in male soccer. *Eur J Appl Physiol.* 108(2): 401–9.

Reilly, T., J. Cabri, and D. Araujo (May 2005). Science of Football V (E1). London, Taylor & Francis Group. Doi/10.4324/9780203412992.

Richard, J.D., A. Chohan, and A. Erande. 2013. *Tidy's Physiotherapy.*

Sale, D. 1986.Neural adaptation in strength and power training. In: *Human muscle power.* Edited by L. Jones et al.: 289–304.Champaign, IL. Human Kinetics.

Sarmento, H., R. Marcelino, M.T. Aguera, J. Campani, and C. Nuno Matos. Dec 2014. Match analysis in football: a systematic review. *J Sports Sci.* 32(20): 1831–1843.

Schache, A.G., T.W. Dorn et al. Sept 30, 2014. Lower-limb muscular strategies for increasing running speed. *J of Orthopaedic& Spots Phys. Therapy*: 44 (10): 813–824.

Schmidtbleicher, D., et al. 2014. Long-term strength training effects on change-of-direction sprint performance. *Journal of Strength and Conditioning Research* 28 (1): 223–31.

Schmidtbleicher, D. Sept. 21. 2019. *Strength training: structure, principles, and methodology.* Strength and conditioning education center. Poland.

Schoenfeld, B.J. 2012. Does exercise-induced muscle damage play a role in skeletal muscle hypertrophy? *Journal of Strength and Conditioning Research* 26 (5): 1441–53.

Seitz, B.L., A. Reyes et al. 25 July 2014. Increase in lower-body strength transfer positively to sprint performance : A systematic review with meta-analysis. *Sports Med.* (44): 1693–1702.

Schmidtbleicher, D. Sportliches Krafttraining und motoriche Grundlaagenfochung. In the W. Bergen et al. 1984, 2019.

Sharma, K.D. and P. Hirtz. 1991. The relationship between coordination quality and biological age. *Med. Sport* 31: 3–4.

Shedler, S., F. Tenelsen, L. Wich & T. Muehlbauer. Nov 2020. Effects of balance training on balance performance in youth: role of training difficulty. *BMC Sports Science Medicine and Rehabilitation*. Doi. 10.1186/s13102-020-00218-44.

Silva, J.R, ,G.P. Nassis, and A. Rebelo. 2015. Strength training in soccer with a specific focus on highly trained players. Sports Medicine-Open. 02 April.

Thorpe, R.T., G. Atkinson, B. Drust, and W. Gregson. 2017. Monitoring fatigue status in elite team sports athletes: implications for practice. *Int J Sports Physiol Perf.* 12:S227–34.

Udofa, A., L. Ryan, K. Klark, and P. Weyand. 2017. Ground reaction forces during competitive track events: A motion-based assessment method. *Int Soc of Biomech in Sports*: 36 (2017) Iss 1.

Van Someren, E.J.W. 2006. Mechanism and functions of coupling between sleep and temperature rhythm. *Progress in Brain Research*. 153: 309–324.

Volpi, P., G.N. Biscotti, K. Chamari, E. Cena, G. Carimati, and R.N. Braganzzi. Feb 12, 2010. Risk factors of anterior crucial ligament injurie in football players: A systematic review of the literature. *Muscle, Ligaments and Tendons J.* 6(4): 480–485.

Von Lieres, H.C. und Wilkau, N.E. Bezodis et al. 2020 The importance of duration and magnitude of force application to sprint performance during the initial acceleration, transition, and maximal velocity phases. *J sports Sci.* 38 (20): 2359–2366.

Weyand, P.G., et al. 2000. Faster top running speeds are achieved with greater ground forces, not more rapid leg movements. *Journal of Applied Physiology* 89 (5): 1991–99.

Weyand, P.G., R.F. Sandel et al. 2010. The biological limits to running speed are imposed from the ground up. *J Appl Physiol.* 108 (14): 950–62.

Werkhausen, A., N.J. Cronin, K. Albracht et al. April 24, 2019. Training-induced increase in Achilles tendon stiffness affects tendon strain pattern during running. *PeerJ Publishing* Doi.7717/peerj.676.

Zatsiorsky, V.M. 1995. *Science and Practice of Strength Training*. Champaign, IL: Human Kinetics.

ABOUT THE AUTHOR

Tudor O. Bompa, PhD, revolutionized many aspects of Western training methods when he introduced his groundbreaking theory of periodization in Romania in 1963. Dr. Bompa also applied his principle of periodization to the development of strength, speed, agility, and endurance. He has personally trained 11 Olympic medalists (four gold), has served as a training and planning consultant to eight other Olympic and world champions, and as an adviser to coaches and athletes worldwide.

Dr. Bompa is professor emeritus at York University, Toronto, where he has taught courses in training theories. His books on periodization and training methods have been translated into 26 languages and used in more than 160 countries for training athletes and educating and certifying coaches. He has been invited to speak in 46 countries and has been awarded certificates of honor and appreciation from national Olympic committees, ministries of education, and sporting organizations of 31 countries. Dr. Bompa has also been awarded with the honorary title of Doctor Honoris Causa by the Polytechnique University of Timisoara, Romania (2017), and NACA, Alvin Roy for Career Achievements (Las Vegas, 2014)

Credits

Cover and interior design: Anja Elsen

Layout: Anja Elsen

Cover image: © AdobeStock

Interior images: © AdobeStock, unless otherwise noted

Managing editor: Elizabeth Evans

Copy editor: Anne Rumery